"Everything you shared in this book was so on point and relevant. I found myself shaking my head in agreement through most of it. (The rest of the time, I was laughing at the humor!)"
— Susan Keillor, editor

Over-Sixty: Shades of Gray
presents its very own:

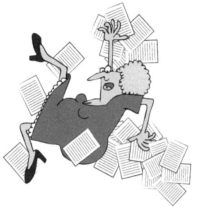

•BOOK
•OF
•LISTS

Barbara Paskoff & Carol Pack

Artiqua Press

www.artiquapress.com

ARTIQUA PRESS
www.artiquapress.com
info@artiquapress.com
Westbury, NY 11590

TRADE PAPERBACK

OCTOBER 25, 2022

BOOK OF LISTS
Over-Sixty: Shades of Gray

ISBN-13: 978-1-970028-11-9

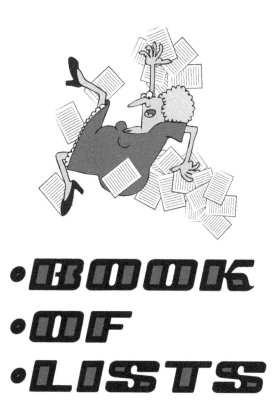

•BOOK
•OF
•LISTS

list

noun

plural noun: lists

1.
a number of connected items or names written or printed consecutively, typically one below the other.

FOREWORD

According to scientific theory, the faster you move through space, the slower time passes.

So, it's just our luck (and yes, we're being facetious) that now that we're over sixty, we've started to slow down—not by choice—and time is whizzing by. The phrase, *So much to do, so little time*, feels appropriate here.

Now if you're anything like us, growing older makes you a bit more impatient, and one of the things you may no longer wish to wade through is a long article promising precious information that could be delivered in a lot less time if the writer used bullet points.

So, here's what this book is about:

- Pertinent information
- Shortened to its essence
- On various subjects

Not to mention:

- Cartoons
- Quotes
- Our own, inimitable, funny little asides

Always.

Need we say more?

Over-Sixty: Shades of Lists
(We wanted to make them gray but they were too hard to read)

TABLE OF CONTENTS

FOREWORD 7

APPEARANCE

Some of us don't care what we look like. These are for the rest of us.

1. Frumpy Is Not Trending 17
2. Beauty Has No Expiration Date 19
3. Here's Looking At You, Kid 21
4. What Wattle? 23
5. Let a Smile Be Your Umbrella 24
6. Twenty-Six Signs You're Getting Older 26
7. My Mirror is Fat 28
8. Hair Today, Gone Tomorrow 30
9. Nailing It! 32

AGEISM

Sometimes it's blatant. Sometimes it's insidious. It's always uncalled for.

10. Ageist Behaviors 36
11. Fifteen Steps You Can Take to Prevent Ageism 38
12. How to Respond to Ageist Remarks 39

ATTITUDE

A positive one can go a long, long way. A bad one will get you more of what you don't want.

13. Accepting the Unacceptable 42
14. Famous Female Firsts 43
15. Stop Taking Yourself So Seriously 45
16. Ten Best Things About Aging 47

17. Ten Worst Things About Aging 49
18. Let's Really Talk 51
19. Men of a Certain Age 53
20. Say This, Not That 56
21. Remember Etiquette? 60
22. Those Were the Days 63

CLASSICAL GAS
IT'S NOT JUST YOU! We're all blowing the emissions standards.

23. Fifteen Fun Facts About Farting 66
24. Behold the Burp 68

FITNESS
Hup, two, three, four...

25. The Key to the Fountain of Youth 71
26. Dealing with Two Wheeling 73
27. Five to Stay Alive 75
28. Let's Dance 77
29. I Used to Be Able to Smell My Feet 79

JUST FOR THE HEALTH OF IT
Because you're nothing without it, except maybe in pain.

30. Nine Ways to Prepare for Your Doctor Visit 85
31. Building a Doctor-Patient Relationship 86
32. Questions to Ask Your Pharmacist 87
33. Twelve Ways to Fight Sticky Snot & Phlegm 88
34. What to Put On Your Medical ID Jewelry 90
35. His and Hers *Down There* Care 91
36. Things That Help You Poop 94
37. A Real Pain In the Ass 95

38. When Your Nose Drips Like a Leaky Faucet   98
39. What to Pack for a Hospital Stay   100
40. A Bowel Movement – Not A Symphony   102
41. So, You Think You Might Be A Hypochondriac   103
42. New Doc? Questions You need to Ask   104
43. What To Do When Your Friends Say You're Flaky   105
44. Keep Your Teeth   107

THE LIGHTS ARE ON BUT...

Sometimes, all our grey cells don't fire in sequence, giving us that vacant look.

45. Seventeen Ways to Improve Mental Health   110
46. Six Behaviors that Promote Positive Aging   111
47. Simple Ways to Manage Stress   113
48. What Was I Thinking?   114
49. I'm So Confused   116
50. Battling Forgetfulness   118

MEDIC-EASY

Medicare, Medicaid, "Medic, I need a shot...of scotch.

51. Seven Things You Should Know About Medicaid   120
52. What You Should Know About Medicare   121
53. Thirteen Interesting Facts About Social Security 123

PACKING IT IN

With regard to our (and everyone else's) final journey.

54. Funeral Faux Pas?   128
55. Dying to Know About Funerals?   130
56. Twice Dead   132
57. My Casket Look Wish List   135

POTPOURRI
The veritable junk drawer of lists.

58. Fifteen Things They Rarely Tell You About Aging   140
59. What the Stars Say About You   142
60. Late Bloomers – and We're Not Talking Undergarments   146
61. Downsizing Your Home   149
62. Decluttering Your House   152
63. Me Casa? New Casa?   154
64. Senior Stoners   156
65. What to Do If Your Passwords Are Compromised   159
66. Regular People Doing Amazing Things After 60   161
67. Why the Old Whore Moaned   162

PRODUCTIVITY
We know; we would rather take a nap as well.

68. You're Retired, Now What?   166
69. Twelve Ways to Fight Boredom   168
70. Procrastination Paralysis   170
71. Picture This   172

RELATIONSHIPS
Until everyone else is dead, you're going to have to deal with relationship dynamics.

72. I do, I did. I'm done. Relationship Deal Breakers   176
73. How to Make Your Mark without a Sharpie   179
74. Aphrodisiacs   180
75. Seniors Helping Seniors   182
76. You're Pissed. Now What?   184
77. Nothing's Like Being a Grandparent   186
78. Teamwork!   189
79. Five Tips to Get You Through the Holidays   191
80. When Your Back Goes Out More Often Than You Do   192

SAFETY
Zip lining does look like fun, but now is not the time to take chances.

81. Nine Nifty Gadgets and Gizmos — 196
82. Twenty-Two Terrific Tips for Aging In Place — 197
83. Must Haves for Your First Aid Kit — 199
84. What to Pack in a Disaster Preparedness Kit — 201
85. Preventing Falls — 203

SELF-AWARENESS
Yeah, yeah, yeah… we get it. But do you?

86. I Smell Old — 206
87. Why Am I Moving So Slowly? — 208

SEX AFTER SIXTY
Does the word "pleasure" mean anything to you?

88. Reasons Why You've Lost That Loving Feeling — 212
89. Sex Toys — 213
90. Ten Ways to Reignite Passion — 214
91. Avoiding Sex Without Offending Your Partner — 215
92. Womansplaining — 216
93. Six Ways to Satisfy Yourself Sexually — 217

SHOW ME THE MONEY
Cashing in on hobbies, experience or knowledge.

94. Reverse Mortgage Pros & Cons — 220
95. Five Financial Fixes for Seniors — 223
96. Senior Scams — 224

THAT'S ENTERTAINMENT!
Something we all seek.

97.	And the Tony Goes to…	228
98.	Fourteen Books with Older Protagonists	229
99.	Radio Podcasts Geared Toward Older People	230
100.	And the Best Director Oscar Goes to…	232
101.	Fifteen TV Shows That Feature Older People	233
102.	Games People Play	235
103.	And the Oscar Goes to…	237

TRAVEL VIRTUOSITY
Going... Going... Gone!

104.	Before You Go Globetrotting	240
105.	Picky Packing Perfection	242
106.	On the Run Travel Tips	243
107.	You're Driving Me Crazy!	245

IN CLOSING
*Yep. That's O60-speak for **last list**.*

108.	Saying Goodbye in Eleven Languages	249
109.	In Gratitude	250

ABOUT THE AUTHORS   254

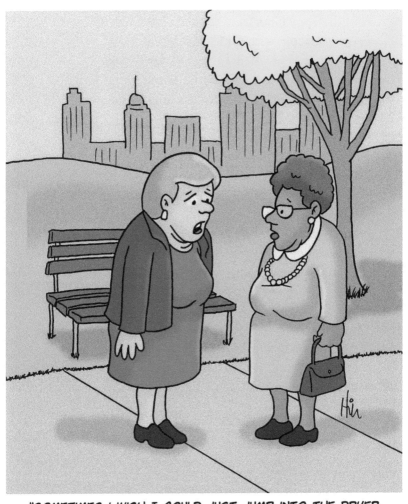

"SOMETIMES I WISH I COULD JUST JUMP INTO THE DRYER AND COME OUT WRINKLE-FREE!"

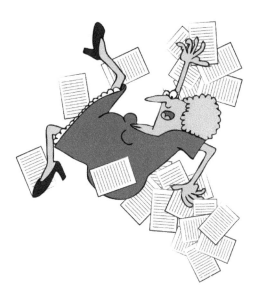

Appearance

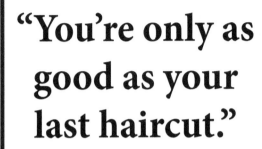

"You're only as good as your last haircut."

—Fran Lebowitz

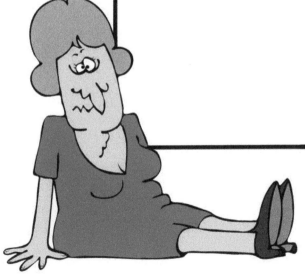

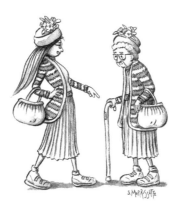

"Where'd you buy that cool cane?"

FRUMPY IS NOT TRENDING

There are fashion DOs, and there are fashion DOO-DOOs:

1. Do wear colors.
2. Do tailor your clothing—make your tailor your friend.
3. Do wear your skirts and dresses at knee length. Many years ago, we used to call a tight-fitting skirt a sheath; now, it's called a pencil skirt. Very flattering. I also like the wrap dress. It looks amazing no matter what body type wears it.
4. Do look for great-fitting jeans. If you have a tummy like me, try shapewear jeans.
5. Do buy a neutral color blazer or jacket that will go with slacks and jeans.
6. Do purchase some tank tops. Who doesn't like a tank (not the kind that would use to mow down your neighbor's favorite magnolia tree)? These tanks go under the blazer you bought.
7. Do keep your accessories at a minimum. When it comes to jewelry—less is more.

8. Do wear well-fitting undergarments. You may need professional advice when buying a bra.
9. Do look for ¾-length sleeves (and sweat like hell in the summer) if you're self-conscious about your arms.
10. Do make sure to have fun shopping, and wear whatever you have on confidently. Posture is essential!

On the flip side:

11. Don't wear clunky shoes (unless your orthopedist demands them).
12. Don't wear baggy anything except pajamas.
13. Don't wear anything too short or too long.
14. Don't dress young. What you wore then is not what you should wear now.
15. Don't show a lot of skin unless you look like Bo Derek.
16. Don't do matchy-matchy (OR ITCHY-ITCHY).
17. Don't be afraid to break the rules if doing so will boost your confidence. No fashion trend is better than confidence.

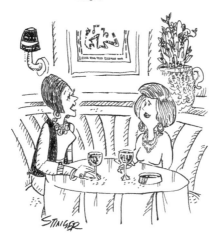

" I'll grow old gracefully when I want to and not any sooner!"

BEAUTY HAS NO EXPIRATION DATE

I just saw #beautyhasnoexpirationdate—and I really believe that message. So, I put together a list of what wise and gentle women can do to retain a beautiful appearance.

- Drink plenty of water
- Stay out of the sun
- Use sunscreen
- Eat a lot of green, leafy vegetables
- Moisturize daily
- Exercise
- Use a retinol product before bed (retinol is said to reduce wrinkles and dark spots and brighten complexions)
- Use a hyaluronic product before bed (hyaluronic acid is known for aiding dry skin and reducing fine lines and wrinkles)
- Stay positive

- Consider injectable face fillers like hyaluronic acid or botulinum toxin, etc.
- Speak with a plastic surgeon to see if laser treatments or a facelift would be right for you
- Smile (while you're smiling, your facial muscles pull upward, reducing the appearance of marionette lines, those creases that go from the outside edges of our lips down to our chins, making us resemble the puppet, Charlie McCarthy)

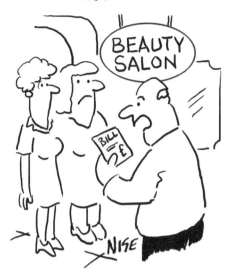

This bill's not a pretty sight either

HERE'S LOOKING AT YOU, KID

Our legs may look like a roadmap (blame gravity and weakening veins), but our faces don't have to.

How?

- If you smoke, stop.
- Eat clean and hydrate.
- Bleach your teeth.
- Go for more of a natural make-up look. Use concealer, and wear lighter lipstick shades. Skip the heavy dark makeup.
- Face powder is a no-no if you don't want to highlight your wrinkles.
- Try a shorter hairstyle. Try some highlights, and don't tease your hair to beehive heights.
- Shape your brows; try to remove excess facial hair. And yes,

21

look up your nose to see if any hairs are ready to emerge.
- Incorporate a skincare routine.
- Try to get facials if they're in your budget.
- Exfoliate. You can make your own scrub by mixing sugar or salt with moisturizer or olive oil, gently massaging it onto your face for a minute or two, then rinsing. Moisturize again.

And if you're worried about your neck, read the following essay.

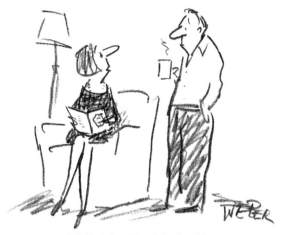

"I feel bad about Nora Ephron's neck."

WHAT WATTLE?

When the late Nora Ephron wrote a book entitled I Hate My Neck, she pretty much epitomized what women of a certain age were all thinking. Turkey wattle doesn't look good on a turkey, so it definitely doesn't look good on us. But we can do a few things to try to minimize its appearance.

- Exfoliate regularly
- Moisturize regularly
- Use a retinol-based neck cream
- Do neck exercises (look up at the sky and open and shut your jaw 25 times a day)
- Posture (hold your head high)
- Eat foods rich in vitamin C
- Take a collagen supplement
- Consider laser skin tightening
- Wear scarves, high collars, and turtlenecks

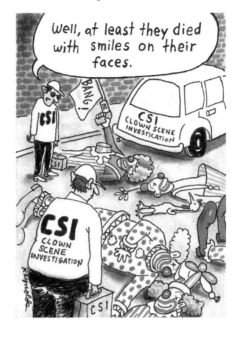

LET A SMILE BE YOUR UMBRELLA

Your smile can change its appearance as you age. The aging process changes the facial structure. The nose (mine got longer and drops into my mouth when I smile) and the jaw can affect how we smile. Not to mention teeth, which shift position due to wear and tear and possible bone loss.

But don't let that stop you from smiling because:

- Smiling is contagious.
- Smiling can make you happier.
- Smiling is attractive.
- Smiling is universal; you don't need a translator.
- Women smile more than men, no kidding.
- Smiling gives you an air of confidence.

- Smiling may give you wrinkles, but it's worth it.
- Babies are born with the ability to smile, and it's not just from a fart.
- Smiling is like medicine; it can reduce your blood pressure, change your mood, and reduce stress.

Not to mention, smiling is easy.

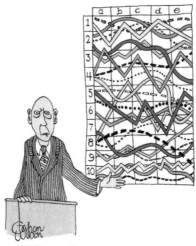

*"I'll pause for a moment so you can
let this information sink in."*

TWENTY-SIX SIGNS YOU'RE GETTING OLDER

A gentleman once told us, "No one wants to be reminded that they're over sixty."

Indeed, many of us act younger and may look more youthful than our actual age. Or we may be in denial. But there are some natural signs that we're getting up there in years. Oh, yes. There are signs.

- Age Spots
- Papery Skin
- More sensitive skin
- Fine lines and wrinkles
- Uneven skin tone
- Visible Pores
- Easily bruised
- Memory problems

- Irregular heartbeat
- Dry eyes
- Dry Skin
- Dry Vagina
- Slower movement
- Weaker muscles
- Less hunger and thirst
- You're shorter
- Less sleep
- More vulnerable to illness
- Digestive problems
- Constipation
- Overactive bladder
- Erectile dysfunction
- Floaters (I used to think they were fruit flies)
- Trouble seeing in dim light
- Hearing loss
- Fatigue

Feel free to add any of your own signs of aging.

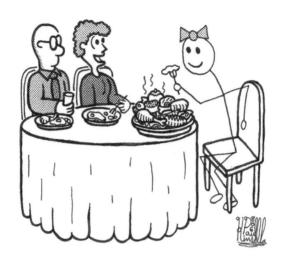

"I envy your metabolism."

MY MIRROR IS FAT

I have an eating disorder. I think it developed in my late teens. Whether it grew from anxiety or low self-esteem, I'm not sure. What I do remember and still experience today is feeling pretty when I'm thin and unattractive if I'm not.

Food is a beautiful thing if it doesn't become your enemy. Truth be told, I shake before I step onto the scale. The number will determine my mood and my food choices for the day. I'm not too crazy about the mirror, either. I don't know if what I'm looking at is real or imagined.

Not everyone with an eating disorder will experience all of these signs and symptoms. It's more of an overview to see if you should talk to a professional.

- Preoccupation with food and dieting
- Not eating specific food groups, like carbs
- Strict calorie counting
- Exercising too much
- Referring to yourself as fat
- Binge eating
- Throwing up
- Skipping meals
- Mood swings
- Feelings of guilt after overeating
- Feelings of poor self-esteem as it relates to your body
- Using laxatives

So, what can we do to help ourselves or a loved one?

- Individual therapy (the most important component of treating eating disorders)
- Group therapy
- Seek the help of a dietician
- A complete medical exam from your primary care physician
- Know you are not alone
- Identify resources in your area
- Contact the National Eating Disorders Association (NEDA) or Families Empowered and Supporting Treatment of Eating Disorders (F.E.A.S.T.).

The National Eating Disorder Association states that approximately 10 million men and 20 million women in the United States will experience an eating disorder at some point in their lives. And more than 20% of adult women 70 and older are dieting and identify weight gain as their greatest concern.

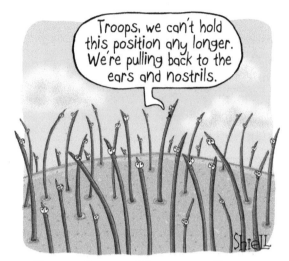

Operation Chrome Dome.

HAIR TODAY, GONE TOMORROW

When we can see more of our shiny scalps than we used to and less shiny hair, there's a reason. Hair doesn't grow as quickly as we get older. Each strand is also more delicate, and our hair follicles produce less of them. We guess you could say they retire.

It could be that we need more hair-producing vitamins and minerals. Or, health-related issues may be causing our tress mess, like:

- Blood thinners
- Chemotherapy
- Antidepressants
- Diabetes
- Hyperthyroidism

Or, if we wear ponytail elastics (guilty), hair clips, or other hair accessories that cause repeated tension in the same place every day, our follicles may have revolted. Then there are the strands that get caught (ripped out!) in the removal of said device.

So, what can we do to protect our tresses?

- Air dry your hair (to prevent heat damage)
- Cut back on chemical treatments
- Choose shampoos that boost strength
- Use hair products that add volume
- Use a silk pillowcase, which allows hair to slide over the surface rather than rub and break
- Use silk scrunchies (gentler on longer hair)
- Use a microfiber towel to absorb moisture rather than vigorously towel drying, which could cause breakage
- Don't wash your hair every day (too drying)
- Gently use a wide-tooth comb or detangling hairbrush on wet hair to avoid breakage

If all else fails, get a pixie cut. Less hair means less stress in maintaining it. We're not talking about shaving your head into a Mohawk (although, if that's your thing, go for it). A pixie cut for older women should be a little softer. Wispy. Short hair doesn't weigh down the face, and wispy bangs can call attention to the eyes and cheekbones while masking forehead wrinkles. The downside is that you must trim it every four to six weeks.

Or try a scalp concealer to disguise bald spots.

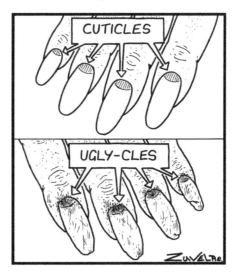

NAILING IT

If you're like me, you've paid so much attention to every other part of your body as it ages that you may have neglected your nails. Or just let your manicurist take care of them. When the pandemic hit, it didn't take long for my acrylics to grow out and my nails to break. I found ridged, cracked nails underneath all the chemicals, and they couldn't grow much past the top of my nail bed without catching on something and ripping apart, sometimes painfully.

What is causing the problem? It could be a number of things.

As we age, our nail growth slows, and they become thicker and more brittle. Blame it on the loss of hormones. That, alone, is responsible for a lot of age-related problems. If you've been relying on acrylics or other products to perfect your nails, perhaps the opposite has happened, and like me, your nails are paper-thin and weak. But the list doesn't end there. The following could also be at fault:

- Using acetone
- Biting your nails
- Low-quality products
- Doing the dishes without gloves
- Your nail file is too harsh
- Vitamin deficiency
- Using your nails to pick staples and scratch-off labels
- Exposure to harsh chemicals

Changes to your nails could also be caused by:

- Anemia
- Hardening of the arteries
- Hormonal issues
- Psoriasis
- Eczema

What can we do?

- Trim fingernails and keep them clean, dry, and filed
- Trim hangnails
- Stay hydrated
- Give nails a day to breathe between manicures
- Moisturize nails and cuticles daily
- Avoid acrylics
- Refuse to use polishes/products containing formaldehyde, toluene, or DBP
- Keep nails on the shorter side
- Wear rubber gloves
- Talk to your doctor

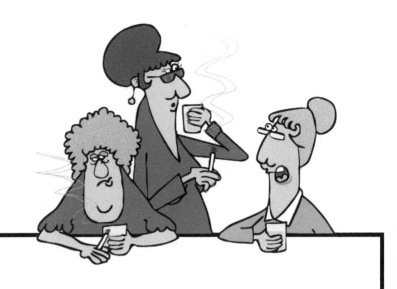

"Some guy said to me:
Don't you think you're too
old to sing rock n' roll?
I said: You'd better check
with Mick Jagger."

—Cher

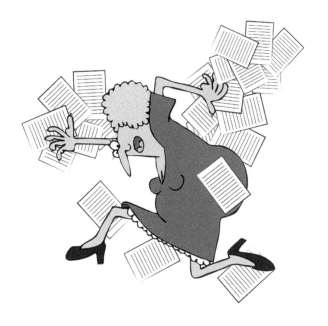

Ageism

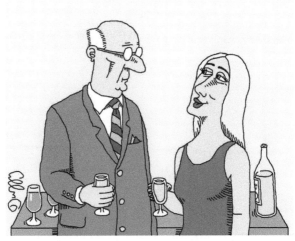

"So, how long have you been old?"

AGEIST BEHAVIORS

We're sure many of us have been the recipient of an ageist remark that has made us feel bad. We can relate to a number of the following:

- People who talk down to you.
- People who stereotype older adults.
- Someone who ignores you because of your age.
- Elderspeak, aka the "we" treatment, i.e., "How are we doing today?"
- Someone who's impatient with you because you're older.
- Younger people who make jokes about senior citizens.
- Professionals who address your children instead of you about your health, finances, or possessions.
- Name-calling, like "geezer," "old bag," or "dirty old man," etc.
- The assumption that older people are technically inept.

- Blaming older adults for social, environmental, or economic problems.
- Treating older adults like children.
- People who "hint" that the elderly should be put out to pasture.

Keep your hopes up. Karma is a bitch. One day, they will be the recipients of the same remarks they're dishing out.

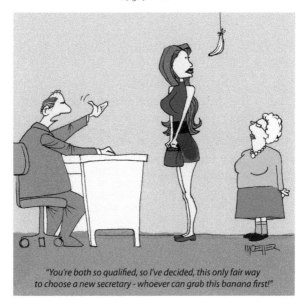

"You're both so qualified, so I've decided, this only fair way to choose a new secretary - whoever can grab this banana first!"

FIFTEEN STEPS YOU CAN TAKE TO PREVENT AGEISM

1. Embrace your age.
2. Have an optimistic attitude.
3. Remain active and aware.
4. Keep up with current events.
5. Engage with others.
6. Identify what you like about yourself.
7. Volunteer.
8. Find a hobby.
9. Do not resist change just because the status quo is familiar.
10. Embrace new technology.
11. Live in the present.
12. Stay independent as long as possible.
13. Mourn what is gone and move forward.
14. Don't allow others to define you.
15. Speak up for yourself.

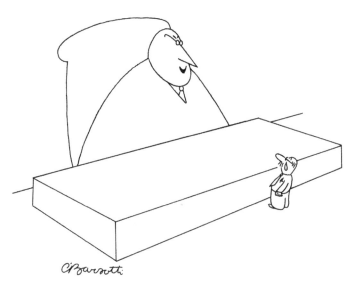

"You're out, Hodges—it's time to make way for a younger loser."

HOW TO RESPOND TO AGEIST REMARKS

This list is how the authors would respond to ageist remarks when it affects us personally.

Barbara likes:

1.   FUCK YOU!

But Carol prefers:

2.   GROW UP!

If you have one of your own, add it here:

3.   _____

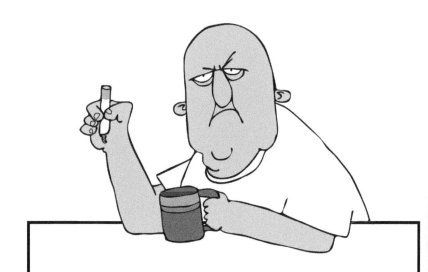

"I'm so old they've cancelled my blood type."

—George Burns

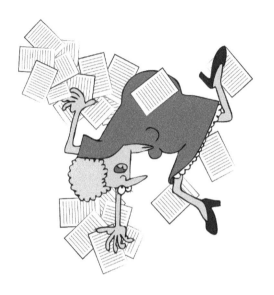

Attitude

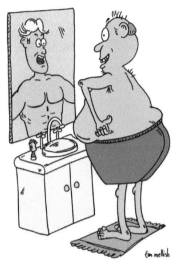

PUSH'N 50, BUT YA STILL GOT IT!!

ACCEPTING THE UNACCEPTABLE... AGING

Try not to let the shame of getting older get in the way of getting older.

- Face reality. It is what it is...until it isn't.
- Try to not let ageist attitudes get to you.
- Embrace the positives: you care less what other people think; blame your *unacceptable* behavior on your age.
- So, you don't feel relevant? Many younger people don't feel relevant.
- Try and lose the words "used to."

You were hot. Now you're not. It's out of your control; move on.

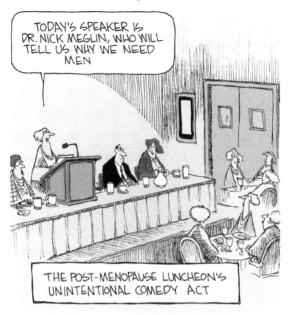

FAMOUS FEMALE FIRSTS

- Kamala Harris – First female U.S. vice president (2021)
- Hattie McDaniel – First African American woman to win an Oscar for *Gone with the Wind* (1939)
- Sandra Oh – First Asian Canadian to win a Best TV Actress Golden Globe for *Killing Eve* (2019)
- Elizabeth Blackwell – First woman to graduate medical school (1849)
- Susan B. Anthony and Elizabeth Cady Stanton – founded the National Woman Suffrage Association (1869)
- Margaret Sanger – Opens first birth control clinic in the U.S. (1916)
- Rosa Parks – Helps start the civil rights movement by not giving up her seat on a bus to a white man (1955)
- Amelia Earhart – Becomes the first woman to fly nonstop across the Atlantic Ocean (1932)

- Betty Friedan – Helps establish The National Organization for Women (1966)
- Billy Jean King – Tennis great, beats Bobby Riggs in the Battle of the Sexes, on primetime TV (1973)
- Sandra Day O'Connor – First woman to serve on the U.S. Supreme Court (1981)
- Sally Ride – First American woman to fly in space, The Space Shuttle *Challenger* (1983)
- Geraldine Ferraro – First vice-president nominee (1984)
- Janet Reno – First female attorney general (1993)
- Madeleine Albright – First female U.S. secretary of state (1997)
- Nancy Pelosi – First female U.S. speaker of the house (2007)
- Edith Wharton – First woman to win a Pulitzer Prize (1921)
- Aretha Franklin – First woman elected to the Rock and Roll Hall of Fame (1987)
- Hillary Clinton – First female presidential nominee (2016)
- Viola Davis – First African American to win an Emmy for Outstanding Lead Actress in a Drama Series (2015)
- Judy Garland – First woman to win Grammy Album of the Year (1961)
- Katharine Graham – First woman publisher of a major newspaper, The Washington Post (1946)
- Marie Curie – First woman to win the Nobel Prize in Physics (which she shared) (1903) and in Chemistry (1911)
- Golda Meir – First female PM in Israel (1969-1974)
- Helen Gurley Brown – First female editor of *Cosmopolitan* who turned it from a struggling family magazine to a sexy handbook for women (1965)
- Eve – need we say more?

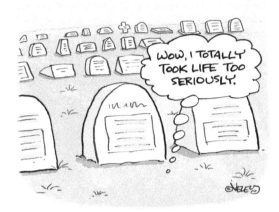

STOP TAKING YOURSELF SO SERIOUSLY

I would bet my last dollar that someone reading this book will know a person who's wound just a little too tightly. They...

- Overthink everything.
- Get anxious or irritated when things don't go their way.
- Dwell on what you would consider the most mundane things (not that I'm being judgy or anything like that).
- Can't accept what they cannot change.
- Try to hide what they consider their imperfections.
- They are afraid to do things out of their comfort zone.
- Point their finger at other people's faults instead of looking inward.
- Can't laugh at themselves. (If I didn't laugh at myself, I'd still be in therapy. Oh, wait! I am.)

Some people are going to like you. Some people are not going to like you. And some people aren't going to give a damn about you. So, be yourself so you can like yourself."

—Dr. Joseph Gyimesi, psychologist

Some reasons for this behavior:

- Fear of rejection and ridicule.
- Anticipation of not pleasing everyone.
- How your parents perceived you.

So, snap out of it. Try the following:

- Let go of what you think your self-image should be, or what people perceive you to be, and just be.
- Push yourself out of your comfort zone so you can grow. Scary, I know. But it builds confidence.
- People being people are going to judge. But that doesn't mean you have to take on their judgment as your identity.
- Keep your expectations within the realm of reality so you are not disappointed in not living up to them.
- Try not to be so easily offended.
- Hang out with funny people.
- Accept your flaws. Or, as I would say, accept yourself warts and all and embrace them.
- Stop overthinking. Sometimes, it is what it is because it just is what it is.

It's been said that "Laughter is the best medicine." No prescription is needed. Just help yourself to a chuckle three times a day.

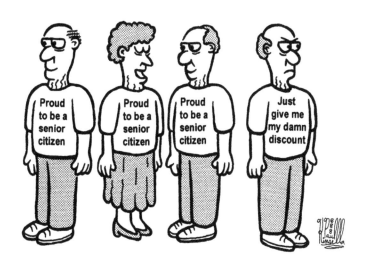

TEN BEST THINGS ABOUT AGING

1. Not caring what other people think.
2. More time to pursue hobbies.
3. Grandchildren.
4. No more PMS—few women ever welcomed monthly menstruation.
5. Wisdom—you've accumulated a lifetime of knowledge and experience.
6. The desire to accumulate material possessions does a 180 degree turn.
7. Not having to wake up to an alarm clock every day.
8. You become less emotional about things happening around you—been there, done that.
9. Life experience gives us a broader perspective.

10. Senior discounts. These are some of the discounts in effect in 2022:

        Amtrak – 10% discount to riders over 65

        Marriott – reduces room rates by 15% or more for guests over 62 who book directly

        Most movie theaters – offer a senior discount

        Burger King – 10% off for 60 plussers

        Dunkin Donut – free donut with large beverage for AARP members at participating restaurants

        Kohls – 15% on Wednesdays

        Cell phones – ask your provider about discounts for seniors

This is just a partial list. Ask about senior discounts wherever you go. Who doesn't want to save money?

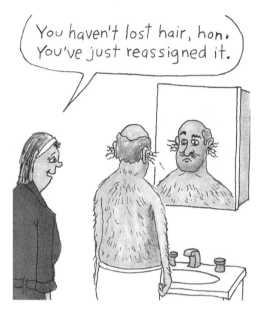

TEN WORST THINGS ABOUT AGING

1. Food doesn't taste the same—whether it's the effect of medication or just that you no longer have as many taste buds, food tastes differently.
2. Hairs grow in odd places, like our ears, nose, or chin, yet thins out where we want them, like on our heads, eyebrows, and eyelashes.
3. Falling down. As we age, we lose feeling in our feet, giving us a greater chance of falling. Not to mention the fear of falling.
4. Self-confidence may decrease after retirement. Many people feel defined by their careers and lose that sense of self after retiring or being replaced at work by a younger person.
5. Ageism. Being ignored, invisible, treated like children—and primarily by younger people with less life experience than we have.
6. We get shorter. Our vertebrae condense. Go figure.

7. Our hands become weaker. Childproof packaging makes products harder to open. Our fingerprints wear down. Objects slip from our grip more easily.
8. Forgetfulness.
9. Time speeds up as we slow down.
10. Painful joints (use a roach clip, so you don't burn your fingers. Oh. Not *that* kind of joint).

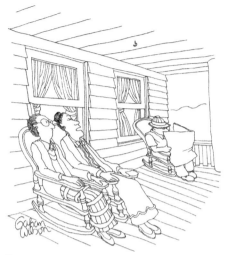

"I always know what Harry's going to say, and he always knows what I'm going to say, so, by and large, we just don't bother."

LET'S REALLY TALK

Please don't assume that because I'm over sixty, I don't enjoy stimulating conversations and hot topics. Or that I don't want to engage in group discussions.

However, I don't know anyone at any age who would want to acknowledge someone who's condescending, gives unsolicited advice, or refers to a person using pet names like honey, sweetie, or sugar.

There is a tendency to presume that all older people are limited. Yes, we are older, we look older, and some of us may act older. However, we are multi-dimensional. Here's what we like to talk about:

• Fun topics

- Existential philosophies
- How often we use the words "used to"
- Drinking (it's five o'clock somewhere)
- Fashion
- Current events (only if it doesn't cause you to lose friends)
- Family
- The assholes we know who are pissing us off
- Theater or the arts in general
- TV shows
- How to pay it forward
- Our wishes and dreams
- Our shrinks
- Restaurants
- Gossip
- Who's doing who
- Our kids
- Our pets
- Book clubs
- Sports
- Hobbies
- Vacations
- High school and college reunions
- Dressing for Zoom calls
- Online seminars
- Any new skill we would like to learn

And this is just for starters!

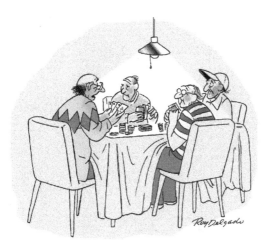

" I'll see your Social Security Supplement and raise you a
Medicare card and a Canadian pharmacy ID. "

MEN OF A CERTAIN AGE

I just asked my husband, "Michael, how old do you feel?"

He said, "Except for my body aches, I feel like I'm in my fifties. I do things like I'm in my fifties. I just can't move like I'm in my fifties." Most men we spoke with say they feel the same way.

One noticeable omission from their responses was sex. Not too surprising, considering hormones play a huge role in the aging process. Here are some quality-of-life responses they shared:

Michael P.

- I enjoy reminiscing about the good old days.
- Casinos. I especially look forward to going to Vegas for Super Bowl with my friends.

- Present-day politics and getting angry, which, according to my wife, I excel at.
- Watching and participating in sports. I play tennis twice a week. I could play more, but my knees hurt.
- Going to work. Although I might complain about the BS every so often, working makes me feel productive.
- Going out to dinner with friends.

Donnie G.

- Being with my kids and grandkids.
- Playing golf.
- Working.
- Socializing.

Norman S.

- Playing cards with my friends.
- Eating out.
- Current events.
- Monthly zoom with musicians I've worked with in the Catskills in the '50s and '60s.
- Old-time stories, mostly exaggerated as they are retold over and over.
- Weekly zooms with my cousins from all over the world.
- Keeping up with family matters, health, achievements, etc.
- Monthly networking dinners.
- Golfing and drinking with my buddies, enjoying each other's company, telling old jokes, and making stupid bets.
- At this time of my life, I'm looking to stay healthy enough to continue doing all of the above.
- Things that I never discuss are politics, religion, and children. That will keep me healthier.

Don P.

- I still enjoy being involved in work.
- I enjoy playing golf.
- Being in Florida during the winter, sitting by the pool is terrific.
- Reading.
- And being with my grandchildren.

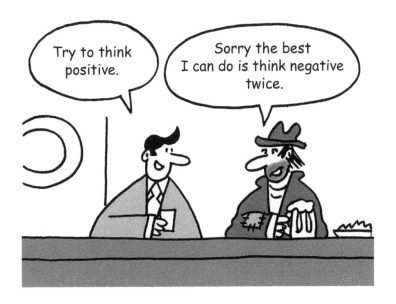

SAY THIS, NOT THAT

"If only I were smarter." "I didn't deserve this award." "I can tell, it's just going to be one of those days." Sound familiar?

Are we aware of how many times during the day we talk negatively about ourselves? This is called self-deprecation. The dictionary defines this negative self-talk as "the act of reprimanding oneself by belittling, undervaluing, disparaging oneself, or being excessively modest."

We often minimize our self-worth during conversations with our friends or business acquaintances. In a social setting, coming across as conceited is a no-no, so putting ourselves down may be an easier route to take to make the people around us feel more comfortable. But at whose expense?

Comedians are known for their self-deprecating humor, and they are hilarious. But we aren't doing stand-up anytime soon.

That's not to say you can't sprinkle a little self-deprecating humor in a conversation every so often, but you don't want it to become an automatic reflex. You know what they say—if you say something often enough, you'll start believing it. If that happens, you may feel more anxious and apprehensive about taking on new challenges. You need to protect your self-esteem and self-perception.

Let's start changing how we choose to frame our responses by putting a more realistic spin on negative thoughts.

NO.　I don't deserve that compliment.
YES.　Thank you. And since you looked so cute saying it, tell me again.

NO.　I can't do this.
YES.　It's intimidating, but I'm going to do what I can. I need to at least try. If I don't, I'll never know.

NO.　Can I be any more stupid?
YES.　I need to do some research.

NO.　I can't deal with the technology.
YES.　I'll take one step at a time, and it will be fine (and then I'll call my grandson).

NO.　I'm too old to try something new.
YES.　I'm never too old to try something new.

NO.　What a dumb thing I just did.
YES.　I will learn from my mistakes. They are lessons in disguise.

NO. I could have done more.
YES. I did what I did, and that's better than nothing. There is a next time. I will do better (I could have done less…).

NO. I'm fat.
YES. To tell you the truth, I'm still working on this one (Marilyn Monroe and I are similarly voluptuous).

NO. I'm so old.
YES. I am lucky to have gained wisdom through living my life. I am thankful for lessons learned (the longer I live, the more birthday cake I get to eat).

NO. Damn, I should have won.
YES. Being in the race shows courage. I will apply myself and work harder the next time around.

NO. I hope I don't fuck up.
YES. My past accomplishments have always been challenging, but I've always managed to get through them.

NO. I don't have the talent.
YES. I am talented in so many other areas. Why concentrate just on this?

NO. I'm loud.
YES. I have a large personality. I'm unique. (Turn down your damn hearing aids.)

NO. I don't fit in.
YES. I have a wonderful relationship with my family. I fit in just fine.

NO.   I Can't remember shit!
YES.   Just having one of those days; some memories are better than none.

NO.   I just can't get organized.
YES.   I need to just take one step at a time.

NO.   I'm just boring.
YES.   I don't have to be entertaining all the time.

NO.   I'm lazy
YES.   I'm unmotivated right now. (I've earned the right to relax. Just ask the government. They call it retirement.)

NO.   I wish I had blah blah blah…
YES.   I am grateful for the little things. You know what they say: "The best things in life are free." (Which is why so many thieves enjoy free room and board in our state prisons.)

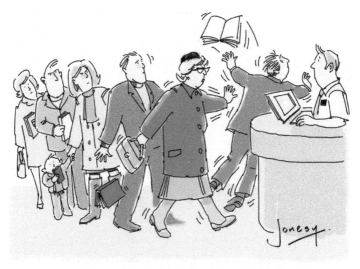

"I'm looking for a book called 'The Decline of Manners' by A. S. Thorpe."

REMEMBER ETIQUETTE?

When I was a little girl, I remember sitting with my father at the dinner table and writing thank-you notes to my parents' friends who had given me gifts. It was our ritual. I would get a gift, he would ask if I'd written a thank you note, and if I didn't, he would sit me down, hand me a pen and a piece of stationery, and wait until I finished.

Even if email had existed way back then, he would still have insisted on a handwritten note.

From rotary telephones to technological advances to wearing only black at funerals, much has changed since the original publication of Emily Post's book on etiquette.

Life was slower then. More formal. Perhaps even more considerate. Today we find ourselves rushing to get from point A to point B. Does anyone have the time to hold the door open for the person behind them? Let's see.

Then and now:

Then: Dressing up to go on a plane.
Now: Wearing what's comfortable, as long as your crack isn't making a public appearance.

Then: Soothe a male ego no matter what.
Now: I don't think so!

Then: Men took care of women in public by helping them with their coats and standing up when they entered the room.
Now: Don't hold your breath.

Then: Men opened doors for women.
Now: Yes, they should, and we should also hold the door for them.

Then: Men were expected to pay the bill.
Now: Make your arrangements before the check arrives.

Then: Women should not shake hands.
Now: Shake hands. Do a fist bump. Do an elbow bump. Do a butt bump.

Then: No elbows on the table.
Now: Where else would they be if you want to keep your balance while reaching your fork into someone else's dish.

Then: Returning phone calls.
Now: Text or email.

Then: Ladies first.
Now: First come, first serve (so why aren't you serving me?)

Then: No one spoke on the phone at the table.
Now: Everyone speaks on the phone at the table.

Then: No white after Labor Day.
Now: Hmn. What if you're a bride?

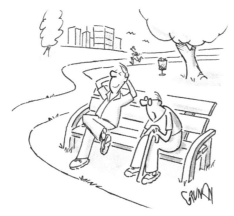

"What 'good old days'? You must have missed the Depression and World War II."

THOSE WERE THE DAYS

- When I had a full head of hair
- When I had one chin
- When my thighs didn't rub
- When my legs didn't look like a road map
- When I had to shave
- When my nose was smaller, and I was taller
- When I had one stomach
- When I could bend down with straight legs
- When my complexion was free of freckles...large freckles
- When I woke up after a good night's sleep without pains
- When I could taste the full flavor of what I was eating
- When my underwear, at the end of the day, was fresh as new
- When my eyes, vagina, and skin weren't dry
- When my skin and nails weren't so brittle
- When I could hear without tilting my better ear in the direction of what I was trying to hear
- When being on a diet showed results

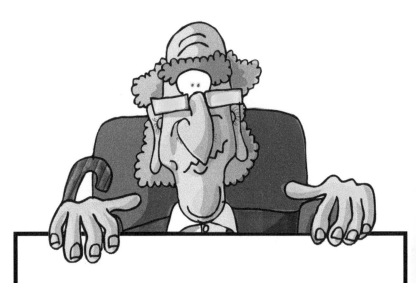

"Fart for freedom, fart for liberty—and fart proudly."

—Benjamin Franklin

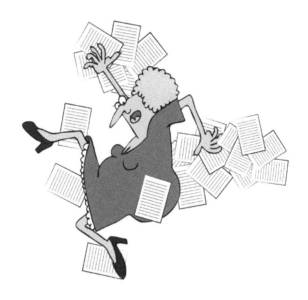

Classical Gas

Seven Dwarfs...
(the later years)

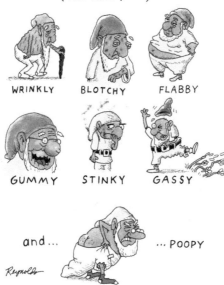

WRINKLY   BLOTCHY   FLABBY

GUMMY   STINKY   GASSY

and...   ...POOPY

Reynolds

15 FUN FACTS ABOUT FARTING

1. Most people fart close to 22 times a day. I fart more.
2. The more you age, the more you fart.
3. Your sphincter weakens as time goes by.
4. Lactose and fructose intolerance, cruciferous vegetables, medications, slower digestion and swallowing too much air are some reasons older folks fart more.
5. A woman's fart smells worse than a man's. According to my husband, "Most definitely."
6. Farts can travel at the speed of 10 feet per second.
7. It's possible farting every day can fill up ½ of a balloon, but getting the gas in there is a bitch.
8. You can light your farts with a cigarette lighter. This is true, my high school boyfriend loved to make me laugh.

9. The rotten egg smell comes from a small percentage of a gas called hydrogen sulphide.
10. A tight ass equals a louder fart. *Makes sense.*
11. The word comes from the Middle English words: *ferten, feortan* and *farten*, and is related to the Old High German word *ferzan*. Fart was coined in the 1600s.
12. You can't spread germs through farting. Consider your underwear an ass mask.
13. Farting can be a turn on. It's called eproctophilia.
14. There are people who fart for a living, they are called flatulists. No, no, not musicians.
15. A dead person can fart for hours after dying.

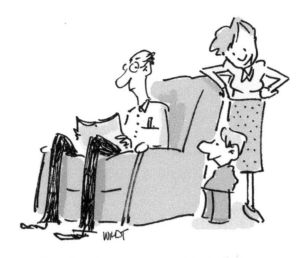

"Well, of course Granddad tweets.
He also grunts, snorts and burps."

BEHOLD THE BURP

- The medical term for burping is eructation.
- Burping is expelling gas through your mouth.
- As you age, you burp more.
- The less you burp, the more you fart.
- The older you get the longer food remains in your system, producing gas.
- Cows in the US burp millions of tons of gases into the atmosphere annually. Ten burping cows can heat a small house.
- The longest burp ever recorded was 1:13 and 57 milliseconds.
- Burping in some cultures is a compliment.
- Some people can burp up to 20 times a day.
- Most animals burp, but not chickens.
- The loudest burp recorded was 109.9 decibels, which is high enough to cause hearing impairment.

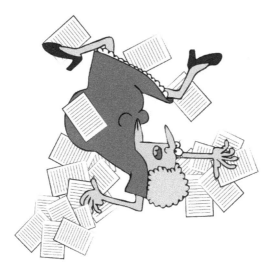

Fitness

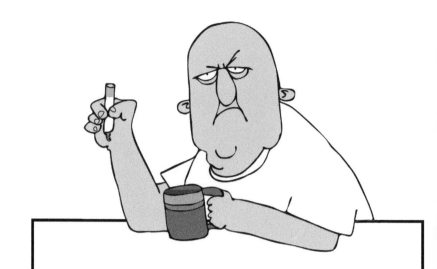

"Sweat is your fat crying."

—Author Unknown

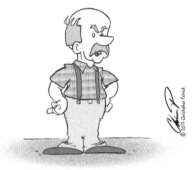

People keep telling me that
it takes more facial muscles
to frown than it does to smile...

I tell them that I'm working out.

THE KEY TO THE FOUNTAIN OF YOUTH

When we were younger, we were quick-thinking, energetic, enthusiastic, sexy, and confident.

Would you like the key to:

- Boosting hormones?
- Building self-esteem?
- Decreasing unhealthy cravings?
- Easing depression?
- Enhancing concentration?
- Improving brain function?
- Increasing your libido?
- Lifting your mood?
- Promoting sleep quality?
- Reducing anxiety?

- Sparking your enthusiasm?
- And raising energy levels?

The one-word answer is *exercise*. It's that simple. Daily physical activity, like walking, can be a magic pill to sustaining overall health. Even seniors who use wheelchairs can do side twists, knee lifts, and use light weights or exercise bands to get a daily workout.

Whoever coined the phrase, "use it or lose it," knew what they were talking about.

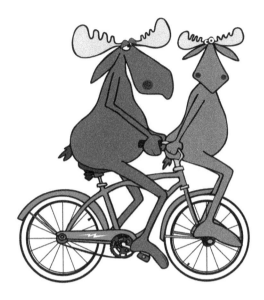

DEALING WITH TWO-WHEELING

Cycling is an excellent outdoor activity that combines fitness and fun, but if you haven't been on a bicycle in a while, there are some things you may want to consider:

- Start small. Feel comfortable and confident before increasing speed, distance, or riding on hilly terrain; get used to the feel of the brakes.
- Ride with traffic, not against it.
- Practice riding with one hand. This will make it easier to use hand signals when turning.
- Wear a helmet. It's for your own protection.
- Brightly colored and reflective clothing makes you easier to see.
- Ensure your bicycle is in good working order: your brakes are operating, and the tires are properly inflated.
- Use the brakes when getting on or off to keep the bike steady.

- Keep your eyes on the road, but be aware of what's happening around you.
- Ride several days a week for fitness.
- Avoid overly ambitious rides until you build endurance.
- Consider packing water and energy bars for longer rides.
- Wear sunscreen.
- Use reflectors if you're riding at night.
- Keep handstands down to a minimum.

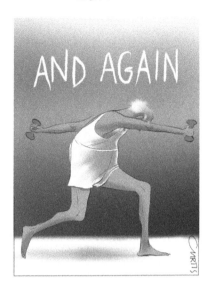

FIVE TO STAY ALIVE

There are five different types of exercise you may want to engage in several times a week to maintain fitness and prolong life.

1. Warm up – this is a must in order to prevent injury. Walking or marching in place is good, but you also want to warm up your mid and upper body with arm circles, shoulder squeezes, and torso rotations. If you break a sweat, that's good because it means your muscles are warm.

2. Aerobic – anything from running to walking, biking or swimming strengthens your heart. If you're like Barbara, you play tennis. Even dancing is aerobic. And if it takes music to make you move, crank up the tunes and shake your booty.

3. Strengthening – squats, curls, lunges, and dips help build strong muscles (just like Wonder Bread). Or climb stairs. Resistance bands and weights are great, too, but lifting cans of soup or bags of groceries also works to build strength.

4. Stretching – there are various stretches you can do to elongate your muscles and make them more flexible. Squats and lunges. Squeezing your shoulder blades together to stretch out your chest. Reaching for the sky or your toes.

5. Balance – holding all your weight on one foot for 30 seconds or more, then switching your weight to the other foot for another 30 seconds will help you build stability and prevent falls.

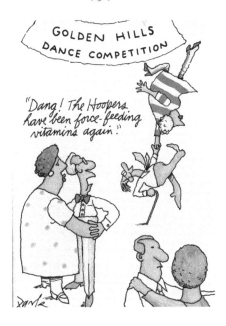

LET'S DANCE

Ballroom dancing has been around for centuries. But it wasn't on my radar screen. A cha-cha-cha and a lindy perhaps at a wedding. But when *Dancing with the Stars* became a thing, ballroom dancing became my go-to hobby.

The dancers were gorgeous, handsome and their bodies, nothing short of perfect. Their athleticism—off the charts.

I've been to a lot of competitions and their senior division, which includes people in their sixties, seventies and eighties, is something to be reckoned with (and they are not out there with their walkers).

Dancing is anything and everything you want it to be. It has an incredibly positive effect.
• It releases stress

- It keeps you feeling young
- It keeps you in shape
- Its athletic aside from beautiful
- It keeps your mind active
- Trying to remember the choreography keeps your brain stimulated
- It challenges you and gives you confidence
- It encourages a social life

So, if you are feeling under the weather and perhaps a little sad, trust me when I tell you it's time to get on the floor and dance your way to happy.

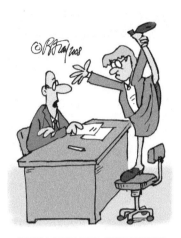

"WHEN I ASKED IF YOU WERE FLEXIBLE,
MRS. HARKNESS, I WAS TALKING
ABOUT YOUR HOURS!"

I USED TO BE ABLE TO SMELL MY FEET

Remember the days when you could touch your toes with your fingertips? Or be able to do splits? Or be able to pick your leg up to your nose and smell your feet? Ah, how easy that was then. Today not so much.

It's an almost done deal that our bodies will lose their flexibility as we age as well as our full range of motion—think soft tissue that surround our muscles, tendons, and ligaments. We need to juice up our bodies, my friends, to stay strong, prevent injuries and remain independent. Regular physical activity will help us accomplish this, and help keep our bones strong. Before you begin any exercise, remember to stretch, and stretch daily. There are more exercises available then the ones listed below.

1. Yoga. I would take yoga later in the day and sleep like a baby.

79

2. Pilates. It saved my back. I had 4 herniated discs.
3. Dancing. Zumba. Really fun. Sweat to the music.
4. Gardening.
5. Swimming.
6. Weightlifting. Me, just getting out of bed.
7. Walking. Easy, breezy.
8. Tai Chi.
9. Massage to release tight muscles and relieve tension.
10. Floor exercises. Push-ups, sit-ups, and lunges; just hope you can get up.

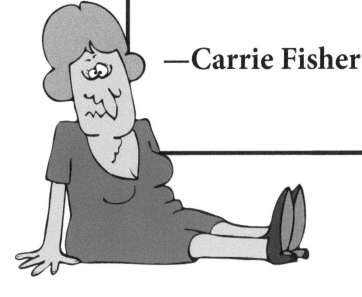

"As you get older, the pickings get slimmer, but the people sure don't."

—Carrie Fisher

81

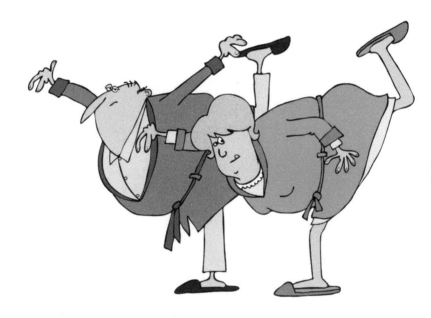

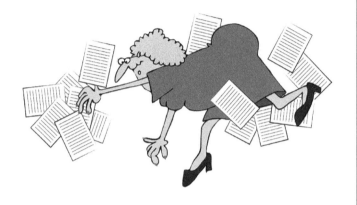

Just for the
Health of It

> "I told my doctor I wanna stop aging… He gave me a gun."

> — Rodney Dangerfield

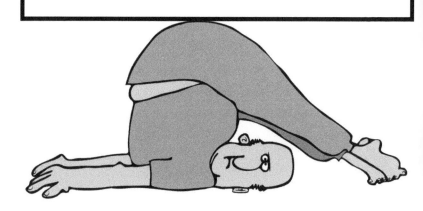

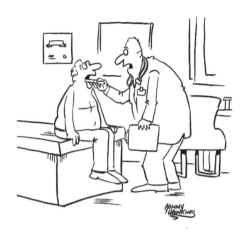

"No, really, it's okay … I was done
with the popsicle."

NINE WAYS TO PREPARE FOR YOUR DOCTOR VISIT

1. Prioritize your concerns, and write down your questions.
2. Bring a pad and pen to take notes if necessary.
3. Ask someone to join you in case something comes up and you need another ear.
4. Bring test results/x-rays and scans with you.
5. If you're having blood drawn, don't eat or drink beforehand. It could interfere with the results.
6. You can also call the office and ask them if there is anything you need to do prior to your visit.
7. Make a list of all the prescriptions you take and the dosage. Include vitamins and over the counter supplements.
8. Learn about tele-medicine.
9. When visiting a new medical professional, it's a good idea to check out the doctor's credentials, reviews, etc.

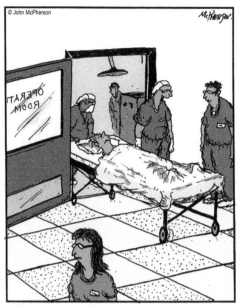

"It was a placebo surgery. I cut him open and just stitched him back up. I guarantee his phantom chest pains will be gone."

BUILDING A DOCTOR-PATIENT RELATIONSHIP

- Your medical history is the major part of your physical exam. Make sure they know everything about you.
- Be honest, even if your questions are embarrassing to you; they have heard it all.
- Be calm and controlled, not controlling.
- Make sure they take the time to answer your questions. Take your own time to think. Don't let them rush you.
- If you feel you're not getting what you need, if the doctor doesn't answer your questions, or if you feel uncomfortable, look for another doctor.

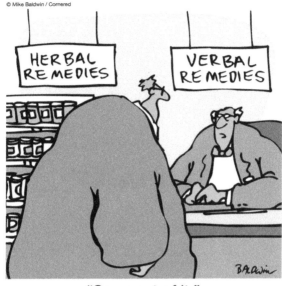

© Mike Baldwin / Cornered

HERBAL REMEDIES

VERBAL REMEDIES

"Snap out of it."

QUESTIONS TO ASK YOUR PHARMACIST

- What exactly is this medication used for?
- What are the possible side effects?
- What drugs or foods shouldn't be taken with this medication?
- How should I take this medication?
- I have allergies. Can I still take this pill?
- Can I stop taking this prescription if I feel better?
- How long has this particular medication been on the market?

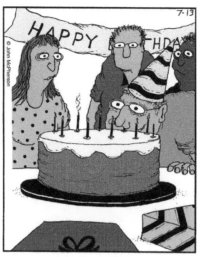

Gary's fondness for snuffing out the candles
on his cake using his nose seriously
dampened the mood at his party.

TWELVE WAYS TO FIGHT STICKY SNOT & PHLEGM

1. Keep the air moist. Your body will fight a dry nose and throat by forming more mucus.
2. Drink plenty of fluids. Staying hydrated thins out mucus.
3. Breathe through a warm, wet cloth. It helps moisturize your nose and throat.
4. Elevate your head, or sleep sitting up. This prevents mucus from pooling in the back of your throat.
5. Cough. It's the body's natural way to remove mucus from your lungs and throat.
6. Spit. When you feel phlegm in your throat, don't swallow it. It's better out than in.
7. Use a saline spray. It will help thin the mucus.
8. Use eucalyptus. If you've ever smelled it, you know it helps congestion.

9. Don't smoke. The body responds to irritants like smoke by producing more phlegm.
10. Try to avoid decongestants. They can make it more difficult to get rid of phlegm and mucus.
11. Avoid inhaling fragrances and irritants. They can make the body respond by producing more mucus.
12. Take hot, steamy baths and showers, or just wash the dishes in hot running water. Steam and hot water can loosen mucus and phlegm.

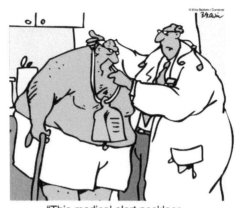

"This medical alert necklace
will help warn people you're approaching."

WHAT TO PUT ON YOUR MEDICAL ID JEWELRY

There is one piece of priceless jewelry we should all own if we suffer from serious health issues. Medical ID jewelry can save your life. Here's what to include:

- Chronic medical conditions like asthma, diabetes, AFIB, etc.
- Medications like blood thinners
- Medical devices like a pacemaker
- Allergies, like sulfa, latex, eggs
- Transplanted or missing organs
- Communication limitations like autism, schizophrenia, hearing impairments
- Do Not Resuscitate orders
- Blood type, if you have a blood disorder
- Contact information

If you're like me, you may need an armful of bling to cover all the bases. Or perhaps I should have it all tattooed across my chest; Lord knows, there's plenty of room there.

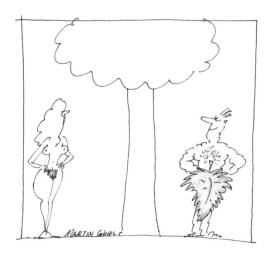

MARTIN GUHL

HIS AND HER "DOWN THERE" CARE

Keeping your vagina and all its parts happy and functioning properly is important work.

Although our pussycat is designed to self-clean with its natural secretions, aging can make it more difficult because of dryness. But all is not lost. There are still a number of things you can do and not do to maintain your vajayjay, starting with a healthy diet and exercise.

- Did you know that the vagina comes in second after the bowel, having the most bacteria? But good bacteria help keep the pH (acid) in balance.
- Wash your vajayjay daily with unscented soaps.
- It is not recommended to douche because it can disturb the normal bacteria and wash out the good stuff inside.
- Scented wipes, sprays, etc., are a no-no. Scented anything, like perfume, should only be sprayed on your neck and wrists.
- After you have sex, if you still do, make sure you pee to avoid

UTIs. And use a condom if you are not in a monogamous relationship.

- Don't shave your pubic hair. It's protective against bacteria, not to mention the itching when it begins to grow in.

As a side note: Many years ago, I was taking a bath and shaving my legs and underarms. What else could I possibly shave? I looked down, and there was my answer. I had plenty to work with, so I shaved my pubes in the shape of a heart for my husband. Happy Valentine's Day!

- Back to dryness. Your car isn't the only thing that may require a lube job. Just be aware that the ingredients you choose should be free of petroleum oils, parabens, scents, and flavors.
- As much as we love to wear fashionable panties, it's best to make sure the crotch is cotton. And try to avoid thongs.
- Give your bottom an airing out and sleep without underwear. That doesn't work for me. I feel naked.
- Check out online sites for sex toys. Not all insertables are safe, so look for ones that are made from stainless steel, stone, etc.
- Practice safe sex.
- See your gynecologist once a year.

Now, for the guys—Penis Preparedness:

There is much more to know about penis health than erectile dysfunction, sexually transmitted diseases, and its ability to help make a baby. And good hygiene is just one of many ways to help keep your penis in good shape.

- It's important that when you wash down there, you wash all the parts.

- "Balls," said the queen. "If I had two, I'd be king." But would she know the importance of keeping them clean and dry? Why? Well, according to the king I'm married to, they need to be powdered up and aired out to avoid infections. Like us females, down there is dark and hidden away.
- Microfiber underwear is best. Boxers are better than briefs for ventilation.
- Use talcum powder with antifungal ingredients daily.
- Use moisturizing soap.
- And if you manscape, just trim to avoid any irritation.
- Practice safe sex.
- See your urologist once a year.
- Get your PSA checked. And no, it doesn't stand for Public Service Announcement. It stands for Prostate Specific Antigen blood test.

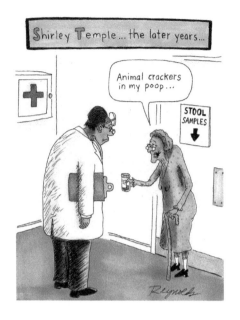

THINGS THAT HELP YOU POOP

- Fiber (broccoli, apples, oatmeal, etc.)
- Fiber supplements
- Water
- Laxatives
- Stool softeners
- Enemas
- Squatting – at our age, our knees may deny us that option, but we can always place a footstool in front of the toilet for our feet to helps us assume the position
- Exercise
- Prune juice
- Hot coffee

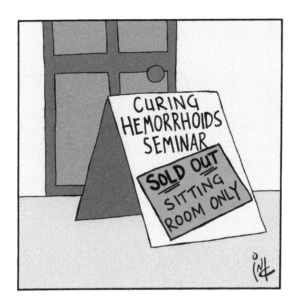

A REAL PAIN IN THE ASS

So, let's talk about hemorrhoids. I have them. Many people I know have them. As a matter of fact, three million people have them. Sometimes they're so painful it's hard to sit. There's the itching. The swelling. The inflammation. And the occasional bleed, which can scare the hell out of you, so go to the doctor and check it out.

Sometimes it's difficult to participate in activities, and that can take an emotional toll.

The only good thing that has come out of this is I'm almost sure my mother wasn't referring to me when she said, "Damn pain in the ass, I wish it would go away."

So, how do hemorrhoids pop up?

- Straining to take a poop
- Reading *War and Peace* on the toilet (too long on the bowl)
- Bouts of constipation or diarrhea
- Engaging in anal intercourse (Ouch!)
- Being pregnant (Aha! Now I know when they began)
- Not watching the scale; getting too heavy
- Eating a low-fiber diet

So, what can we do to hold hemorrhoids at bay?

- As soon as you feel the urge to go, go.
- Drink at least six glasses of water daily.
- Don't squeeze.
- Eat a high-fiber diet.
- Don't take up residency on the toilet.
- Exercise.
- Take stool softeners or fiber supplements.
- After you finish your business, don't scrub the area like you're trying to remove a stain. Use some hygienic cleaning lotion.

Temporary pain relief:

- Sitz bath
- Anal suppositories
- Hydrocortisone for your tush
- Warm compresses

Or you can leave your spouse. Just kidding (not really). My husband agrees!

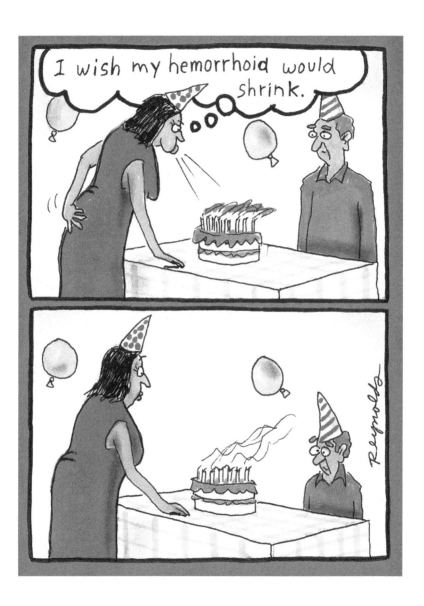

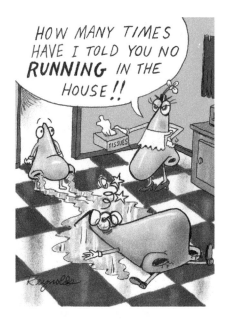

WHEN YOUR NOSE DRIPS LIKE A LEAKY FAUCET

One thing I've noticed as we get older, our noses tend to drip at will with no prior warning. Why?

- Minor temperature changes
- Medications we're taking
- Allergies
- Infections
- Nasal polyps
- Certain foods
- Hormonal changes
- Dust sensitivity
- Age-related changes in our nose structure

Ways to plug the leak:

- Ask your doctor if a prescription can help you.
- Take antihistamines or other OTC medication.
- Reduce clutter at home that can harbor dust.
- Keep windows closed when the pollen count is high.
- Carry extra tissues wherever you go.

Note: Moving to a milder climate may not help because it may have a longer "growing season," meaning a longer pollen season.

Here's looking "achoo" kid!

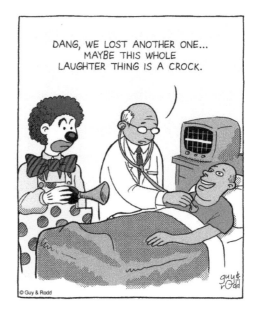

WHAT TO PACK FOR A HOSPITAL STAY

Hospitals provide basic necessities like hospital gowns, toothbrushes, and tissues. However, there are other items you may want to pack to make a hospital stay easier to navigate.

Paperwork:

- Photo ID
- Insurance and Medicare cards
- Applicable reports/scans/pre-certifications by your doctor
- Health care proxy/power of attorney
- Living will
- List/dosages of all medications and supplements you take
- List of allergies, immunizations, chronic and current health problems
- Contact information for family/friends

Comfort:

- Pajamas (must be able to accommodate intravenous lines)
- Bathrobe (must be able to accommodate intravenous lines)
- Sweater (must be able to accommodate intravenous lines)
- Slippers or non-slip socks
- Comb/brush
- Basic toiletries
- Toothbrush/toothpaste
- Eyeglasses
- Dentures and case
- Hearing Aids and batteries
- Books, magazines, crosswords, music for when you're bored
- Paper and pen for taking notes
- A small amount of cash
- Comfortable clothing to wear when discharged

Don't Bother Taking:

- Expensive jewelry
- Portable tech equipment
- Large amounts of cash
- Credit cards
- Checkbook
- Cigarettes or other tobacco products

If you plan to take anything that must be plugged in to operate or charge, check with the hospital first to make sure outlets will be available. Also, keep in mind that small items like watches or wallets, cell phones (if allowed by the hospital), and tablets (if wi-fi is available) can be easily stolen when a patient is incapacitated or sleeping.

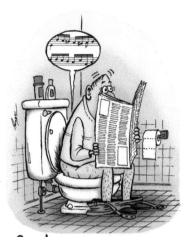

Bowel movement in D minor.

A BOWEL MOVEMENT IS NOT A SYMPHONY

- A normal bowel movement should either look smooth like a snake or crackled like a grilled sausage.
- In the United States, more than four million people have recurring bouts of constipation. While chronic constipation affectsß 63 million.
- An estimated 900 people die from diseases linked to constipation, for example, doo-doo impaction.
- Don't squeeze too hard because you can lose consciousness or faint. I'm surprised I'm still not on the bathroom floor.
- If pooping is challenging, stop eating dairy, meat, sweets, and alcohol. This is enough to depress anyone. Oh, and fried foods.
- If you want to give your bowels a boost, eat fruit, popcorn, nuts, veggies, and prunes; yummy. Keep the fiber and hydration going. I basically live on a stool softener. Sometimes it works, sometimes not so much. Stool softeners help, although they won't soften that hard bench in the hallway.

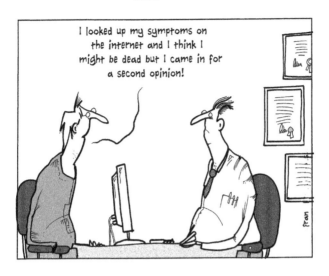

SO, YOU THINK YOU MIGHT BE A HYPOCHONDRIAC?

If you suspect you might be a hypochondriac, take this test:

1. Are you preoccupied with getting a serious disease?
2. Do you worry about minor symptoms, thinking they could be serious?
3. Are you less than reassured after visiting the doctor?
4. Do you spend hours researching the internet for your specific concerns?
5. Are you unable to function because you think you're dying?
6. Do you avoid people, places, and things because you fear a health risk?
7. Do you constantly check your body for signs of lumps, bumps, or other non-specific problems?
8. Are you unable to function because of your fear?

If you answered "yes" to more than half these questions, perhaps you should consider counseling to put your mind at ease.

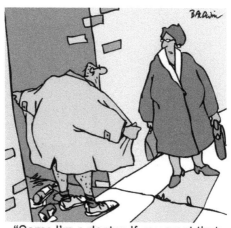

"Sorry, I'm a doctor. If you want that looked at, you'll have to make an appointment like everyone else."

NEW DOC? QUESTIONS YOU NEED TO ASK

When I meet with a new physician, these are some of the questions I ask.

- How long have you been practicing?
- What hospitals do you have privileges at?
- Suppose I need to speak with you right away, how do you handle those calls?
- If you aren't available, then what?
- If a situation arises and you don't know what to do, ask the doctor what he would do himself or recommend for a family member.

Just remember:

- This visit is about you.
- Make sure he's looking at your medical history. It's one of the most—if not *the* most—important parts of your physical.

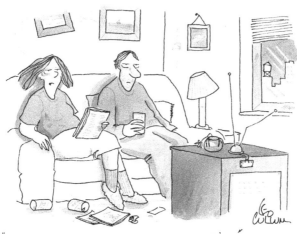

" NINETY PERCENT OF HOUSEHOLD DUST IS DRIED FLAKY SKIN. "

WHAT TO DO WHEN YOUR FRIENDS SAY YOU'RE FLAKY

Older adults can develop dry, rough, or scaly patches as their skin ages. If your skin reminds you of a visit to Aspen, one (or several) of the following reasons may be responsible:

- Not drinking enough liquid
- Spending too much time in the sun
- Cold, dry air
- Smoking
- Stress
- The loss of sweat and oil glands as we age
- Skin products that are dehydrating, like alkaline soaps
- Harsh laundry products
- Hair dyes
- Makeup ingredients
- Adverse reaction to certain medications
- Hot baths

- Skin conditions like eczema or psoriasis
- Systemic illnesses such as lymphoma or malnutrition
- Genetic inheritance
- Chronic illnesses like kidney disease, diabetes or hypothyroidism

So, what can you do to treat it?

- See a dermatologist.
- Use moisturizing creams or ointments twice a day, every day.
- Take warm baths rather than hot ones, and take fewer of them.
- Switch to milder products made for sensitive skin.
- Use a humidifier if the air in your home is dry.
- Avoid products with alcohol or fragrance.
- Wear loose, comfortable clothing that doesn't irritate skin.
- Avoid sitting too close to a fireplace or heat source.

Be kind to your skin. It may not be a Wurlitzer, but it's still your body's biggest organ.

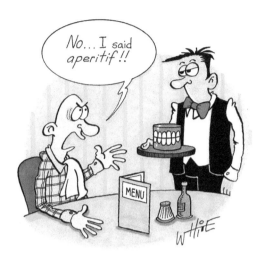

KEEP YOUR TEETH

- Don't chew on ice cubes, hard candy, or gummy candies. The gummy candy pulled a filling right out from my tooth.
- Wear a mouth guard if you play contact sports.
- Wear a mouth guard if you grind your teeth.
- Try and avoid all things acidic. It can wear away your enamel.
- Teeth are not package openers. Use scissors.
- You know that pencil you're using, don't chew on it. Oops, my bad!
- This is not news. Brush your teeth before you go to bed. Also, don't forget to brush your tongue.
- Use mouthwash.
- Drink water.

Just remember: "Lying through your teeth does not count as flossing." —Anonymous

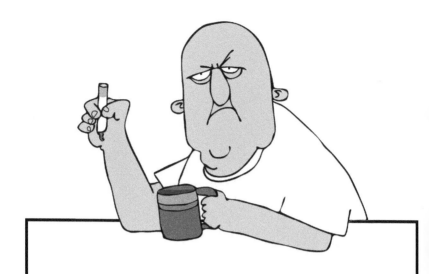

"I always wanted to be somebody, but now I realize I should have been more specific."

—Lily Tomlin

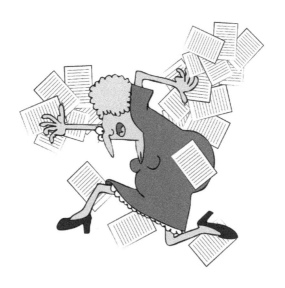

The Lights
Are On, but...

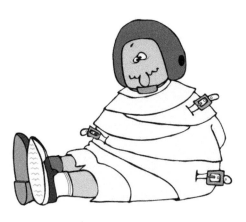

SEVENTEEN WAYS TO IMPROVE MENTAL HEALTH

1. Play mind games to avoid cognitive decline
2. Get physical
3. Stay connected with family and friends
4. Pick up a new hobby
5. Volunteer
6. Care for a pet
7. Join a book club
8. Find a companion with similar likes and dislikes
9. Play a musical instrument
10. Learn a new language
11. Take an art class
12. Share your family history with the youngest family members
13. Write a steamy novel or short story
14. Help fight ageism
15. Join a community theater group
16. Sing in your church choir
17. Play games like mah-jongg, chess, checkers, etc. regularly

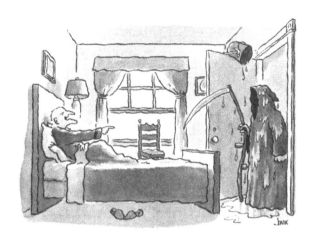

SIX BEHAVIORS THAT PROMOTE POSITIVE AGING

If you're anything like us, you may wake up in the morning feeling less than your usual, ravishing self. It takes us time to get our mojo going. But we've got ways to get your ass moving.

1. Have a goal or purpose when you wake up in the morning. Give yourself a reason to get out of bed.
2. Move. It doesn't have to be exercise. But everyday activities like gardening, riding a bike, or dusting cobwebs keep your blood flowing and prevent you from becoming too sedentary.
3. Relax. You've earned the right to take naps or sit down with a cup of tea, especially if you're stressed. If you feel tightly wound, take the time to unwind.
4. Less meat, more veggies. Eating a greater amount of plant-based foods and stopping before you're completely full will help you control your weight and avoid feeling sluggish.
5. Surround yourself with family and friends. There's nothing like love and support.

6. Laugh. Laughter helps you relax, can boost the immune system, and increase oxygenation in the blood. It also burns calories. Need we say more?

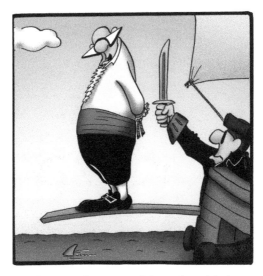

"Do you have any idea what this is
doing to my high blood pressure
right now?"

SIMPLE WAYS TO MANAGE STRESS

1. Slowly sip a cup of herbal tea.
2. Put on your favorite song and just move. Dance, sway, wave your arms, just react as the music takes over.
3. Recall a happy moment in your life and enjoy the memories it sparks.
4. Straighten out your desktop or tabletop. Decluttering something small can help re-establish your feeling of control.
5. Try a breathing exercise: Focus your thoughts on inhaling to a count of four, holding it in for a count of four, then exhaling to a count of four.
6. Get a massage.

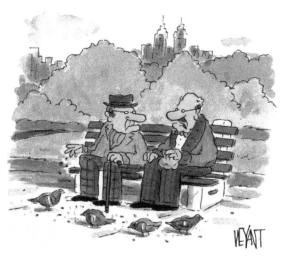

"Just when I thought I had all the answers, I forgot what the questions were."

WHAT WAS I THINKING?

We have all probably walked into a room at one point in our lives and forgotten why we did. It's exasperating, but is it a problem? It depends. Here are some of the causes of forgetfulness.

• Medications: Ask your doctor or pharmacist if the meds you're taking could affect your memory and if so, is there a viable substitute you can take?

• Vitamin deficiency: Too little Vitamin B12.

• Lack of sleep: We're all off our game when we don't sleep deeply enough or long enough.

• Alcohol: It not only lowers our inhibitions, it screws around with our short-term memory.

• Anxiety: There are only so many things we can worry about at

114

once. And it's hard to remember new thoughts when our brains are already occupied.

- Underactive thyroid: An underactive thyroid can be the root cause of several problems, which can lead to forgetfulness, be it lack of sleep or the medication you take for it.

- Depression: The sadness and feeling of hopelessness that comes with depression can cause a lack of focus, resulting in forgetfulness.

- Trauma: Head injury or stroke.

- Work-related stress: Need we say more?

- Chronic diseases: Alzheimer's disease, dementia, brain tumor.

- Aging: Yep. Being forgetful is a common side effect of aging. It usually happens gradually.

If your forgetfulness is sudden or progresses rapidly, you may want to see a medical professional to determine the reason because there are other possible causes.

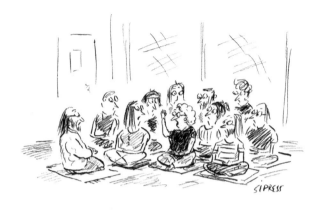

With everything else I've got on my mind, now you're telling me I have to think about breathing?

I'M SO CONFUSED

What do dictionaries say about confusion?

con·fu·sion (kun-fyoo-ZHen) n.
The state of being bewildered or unclear in one's mind about something.

You may experience:

- Brain fog (feeling sleepy or withdrawn)
- Difficulty concentrating
- Irritability (being nervous or agitated)
- Feeling anxious or overwhelmed
- Feeling pulled in two different directions
- Memory lapses

Possible Causes:

- Dehydration
- Medical conditions – like an infection (respiratory, UTI, sepsis)
- The medications you are taking
- Serious illnesses like dementia, Alzheimer's, or Parkinson's

What you can do about it:

- Slow down.
- Breathe.
- Change your focus. Think about something totally different that you know well.
- Use the 5 4 3 2 1 grounding technique:

    5. Look for five things you can see (the sky above, your skin color, the paint on the walls…).

    4. Describe four things that you feel (your waistband, the arms of your chair, gravity…).

    3. Name three sounds you can hear (the whir of an air conditioner, music, birds chirping…).

    2. Pick out two odors you can smell (the cologne you're wearing, something cooking, someone's body odor…).

    1. Identify one thing you can taste (this morning's breakfast, mouthwash, chewing gum…).

- Concentrate on what you can trust.
- Go with your gut.
- Seek additional information about what is confusing you.
- Give yourself the benefit of the doubt.
- Ask for help.
- Write down how you're feeling and what you think is making you feel confused.
- Be patient with yourself.

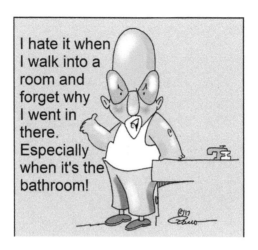

BATTLING FORGETFULNESS

How can you prepare yourself to battle the more common causes of forgetfulness? By taking care of yourself.

- Socialize
- Do puzzles and mind games to keep your brain sharp
- Daily physical activity increases blood flow to your brain
- Get enough sleep
- Eat a healthy diet
- Simplify your life
- Post-It notes!

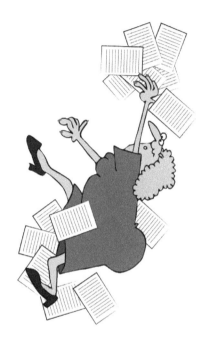

Medic-Easy

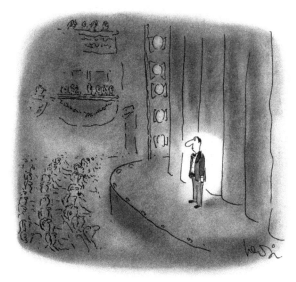

"Is there a doctor who accepts Medicaid in the house?"

SEVEN THINGS YOU SHOULD KNOW ABOUT MEDICAID

1. It's a national health insurance program for low-income folks.
2. Eligibility requirements vary by state.
3. It's not just for "old" people.
4. Medicaid covers one in five Americans.
5. Medicaid provides for services in the home, allowing eligible recipients with disabilities to live independently rather than in institutions.
6. Medicaid is jointly administered by states and the federal government.
7. Some people are eligible for both Medicaid and Medicare.

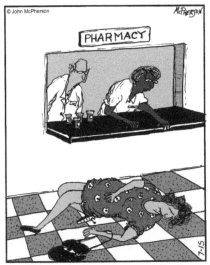

"She's going to need a prescription for light-headedness. She fainted when I told her how much her meds cost."

WHAT YOU SHOULD KNOW ABOUT MEDICARE

We went to the source for these bullet points: www.Medicare.gov.

• Some people get Medicare automatically, and some have to sign up. You may have to sign up if you're 65 (or almost 65) and not getting Social Security.
• There are certain times of the year when you can sign up or change how you get your coverage.
• You can avoid a penalty if you sign up for Medicare Part B when you're first eligible.
• You can choose how you get your Medicare coverage.
• You may be able to get help with your Medicare costs.

But what is Medicare? Like the old commercial used to say, "Parts is parts," and Medicare is made up of parts.

Part A - covers hospital expenses, ambulance services, and skilled nursing home and hospice care.

You usually have to pay a deductible and copayments.

Part B - covers doctor visits, preventive care and lab services, physical therapy, health screenings, vaccinations, and medical equipment.

You will be charged a premium. In most cases, you will pay 20% of the Medicare-approved amount for the service and any deductibles.

Part C - Medicare Advantage Plans cover parts A and B and can include additional benefits like hearing, vision, and basic dental coverage.

You will have to pay your Part B premium as well as the premium for the Advantage plan you select.

Part D - is prescription drug coverage to help with the cost of medications. There are many different drug plans that differ from state to state, and each plan covers specific drugs.

You will have to pay for the prescription drug plan you choose as well as a deductible and co-pays.

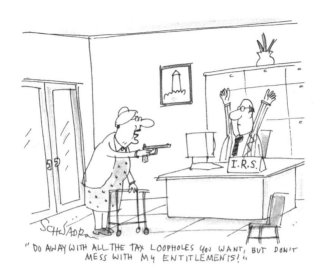

"DO AWAY WITH ALL THE TAX LOOPHOLES you WANT, BUT DON'T MESS WITH My ENTITLEMENTS!"

THIRTEEN INTERESTING FACTS ABOUT SOCIAL SECURITY

1. Social Security was signed into law in 1935.
2. It not only protects retirees but also benefits their spouses and young children.
3. About 15% of recipients are disabled workers between 21 and 64.
4. Uncle Sam will tax your social security benefits if your earned income exceeds a threshold amount.
5. Thirteen states tax social security benefits.
6. Social Security keeps up with the cost of living (in its own way).
7. Your benefit payment is based on what you paid into the program.
8. Social Security benefits are modest, with the average retirement benefit in 2020 being just over $1,500.00 (which is why you should buy one of those houses for a buck in Italy, which has one of the best benefit payouts).

9. If it weren't for social security, millions of older Americans would live in poverty.

10. It takes ten years of work to qualify for social security.

11. You can take a reduced social security benefit as early as age 62, however, the longer you wait to take it, the more the monthly payment will grow until you reach age 70, and it could affect your final maximum benefit by as much as 30%.

12. You can claim social security benefits earned by your ex-spouse as long as you were married for ten years, are 62 or older, and are single.

13. Do-over! If you applied for early retirement, Social Security will give you up to a year to change your mind, as long as you pay back the benefits you received.

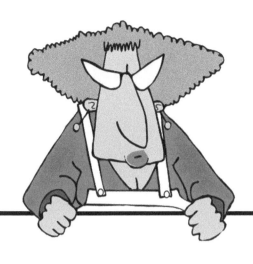

"I'm too young for Medicare and too old for women to care."

— Kinky Friedman

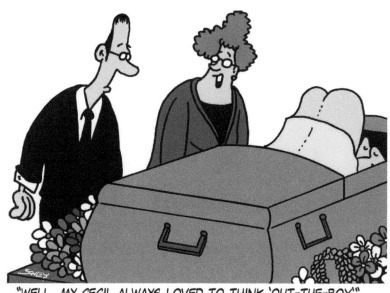

"WELL, MY CECIL ALWAYS LOVED TO THINK 'OUT-THE-BOX'."

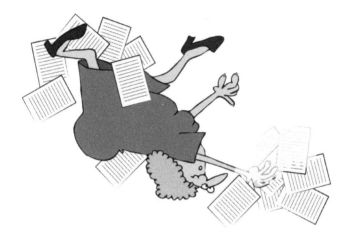

Packing
It In

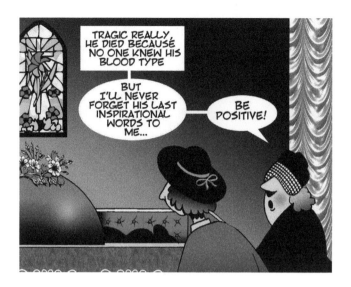

FUNERAL FAUX PAS?

Dropping dead anytime soon is not on my to-do list. And neither are funerals, for that matter. What to wear? What to say? How to behave? How to feel? It's just a dark, lousy moment!

True stories told to us by others:

- "During my grandfather's funeral, my brother and uncle were standing close to the coffin when my uncle said to my brother, 'Don't date anyone outside the religion; Grandpa is going to roll over in his grave.'"

- "I wore white to my father's funeral and red to my mother's."

- "The person conducting the service totally mispronounced the deceased's name."

- "I'm going to wear black because I look thinner."

- "It's okay to laugh and smile. I have a joke. Have you heard the one about…?"

- "Can you imagine someone saying it could be worse? They've said it. Response. 'Yes, he's still alive.'"

And whatever you do, don't take a selfie in front of the casket. "Smile!"

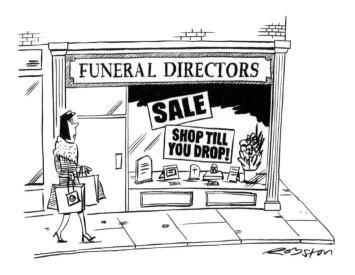

DYING TO KNOW ABOUT FUNERALS

Did you know that when someone dies, their hearing is the last thing to go? I don't know at what point hearing ceases, but let's say it takes a while. So be careful…

- Gravesites are reportedly six feet deep to help prevent farmers from accidentally plowing up bodies and to prevent theft.
- Caskets can be rented.
- Some funeral directors live in the funeral home—a fun house.
- Embalming is not required by law.
- You do not need to hire a funeral director. Just make sure whoever is leading the service knows what the hell they're doing.
- There isn't a coffin on the market that will preserve a body.
- Wearing black goes back to Roman times (Harry L. Marks).

- You can hold a funeral service at any location (golf course, beauty parlor, an amusement park).
- A gravesite does not expire after purchase.
- Some graves are on a hill for drainage.
- Ninety percent of funeral homes are privately owned.
- According to the National Directory of Morticians, there are over 18 thousand funeral homes in the United States.
- As of 2020, the average funeral cost was approximately eight thousand dollars.
- Taberger's safety coffin was developed in 1829. It included a bell to ring, which would alert the graveyard workers if someone was being buried alive (or taking a nap).

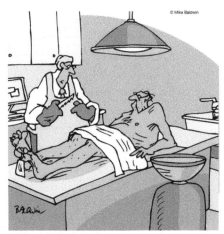

"It's a little late for a second opinion –
this is the autopsy."

TWICE DEAD

The only sure things in life are death and taxes, but taxes are more reliable.

I say that because each of my parents died twice. I know it sounds ridiculous, but it's true. My mother was involved in a fatal automobile accident and was declared DOA when she arrived at the hospital. They covered her face and pushed the gurney to the side. If a passing surgeon hadn't heard her moan, she probably would have died before she ever got to the morgue. He saved her life and gave her another ten years. She was still relatively young when she died the second time—only 68, but that time there was no return ticket.

My father dropped dead on my brother's driveway when he was 78 years old. It was Christmas Eve. My brother had walked inside

132

with an armload of presents, and when he went back outside for more, he found my father on the ground with no pulse. My brother performed CPR for several minutes before my father re-animated (for lack of a better word). Dad spent the holidays in the hospital because it's apparently not a good time to schedule a defibrillator and pacemaker. But once he did get all hooked up, he lived another ten and a half years.

"So, where's the list?" you ask. It's here. If you want to live multiple lives:

- Hang out with people who know CPR.

- After 60, see a cardiologist regularly, and don't balk if he suggests hardware.

- If you're religious, pray that you'll have an angel on your shoulder if and when anything happens to you.

- One of those "fallen and I can't get up" gizmos may not be a bad investment.

- Don't wait until after you've died to tell someone you're sorry or forgive them for past transgressions. Most departure tickets only get punched once.

If you do come back, live every day like it's your last. I don't know anyone who's come back twice. Honestly, if it were possible, my mother would have figured out how to do it.

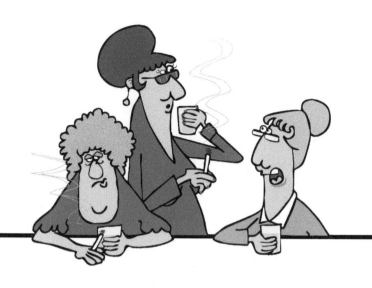

"No matter how great a man is, the size of his funeral usually depends on the weather."

—Rosemary Clooney

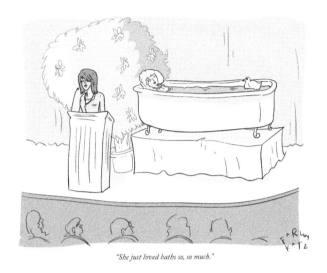

"She just loved baths so, so much."

MY CASKET LOOK WISH LIST

I've told my friend time and time again that if I decide to have a funeral, I want a big one. Huge! A real emotional send-off.

I've taken care of almost everything; the chapel, the cemetery, and my satin-lined casket (I'm thinking a soft blue). But since the *when* is up in the air, *Save the Date* notices are moot.

Now I must get down to the nitty-gritty of how I want to be laid out. My wardrobe, hair, and makeup need attention. I want to look drop-dead gorgeous.

I will have hired a makeup artist and assistants. The directives:

- Full face makeup. Eyelashes, eyeliner, eyeshadow. A shimmering blue would look nice and coordinate with the silk casket lining. And a self-tanner because I don't want to look too gray.

135

- I will wear my red Michael Kors dress that I bought years ago at the outlet. I love me a good bargain. No jewelry. Gave all of it to my daughter.
- As far as my hair is concerned, I think a ponytail is just fine. I've been losing so much of it over the years, anyway. I'll just have them tease what's left for volume.
- A sweater for the change of seasons.
- No religious speak.
- I want to be buried with my dogs' ashes.
- Gifts for the guests as they leave the service. I haven't decided yet on what.
- And for those who are dying for a cup of coffee and a nosh before the schlepp to the cemetery, a dessert wagon will be parked in front of the entrance as you walk to the parking lot.

Please no flowers; instead, donate to the charity of your choice.

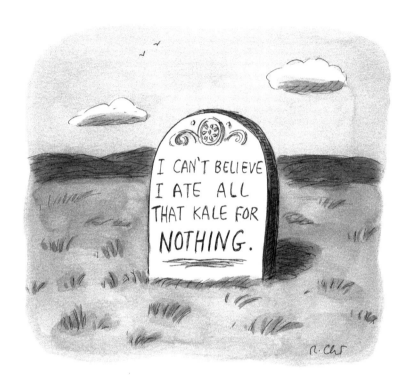

137

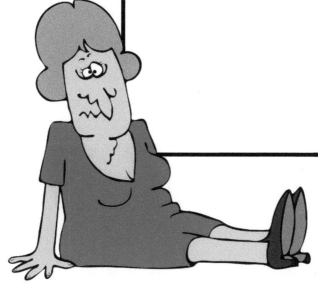

"Wherever you go, there you are."

—Confucius

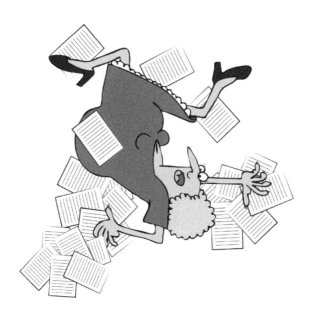

Potpourri

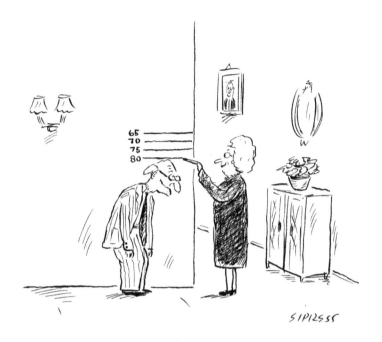

FIFTEEN THINGS THEY RARELY TELL YOU ABOUT AGING

1. We shrink—not just in height, but our brains shrink as well. Not to mention penises and testicles.
2. Our sleep patterns change. We fall asleep. We're up. We're still up, but maybe we'll fall back to sleep. If we're lucky. And that's just during the day.
3. We can develop adult acne. I did at 30.
4. Our skin is thinner. Collagen breaks down, making skin more susceptible to bruising. Think road map on your legs.
5. Body temperature changes—we're not feeling the heat as much, but we are feeling the cold.
6. Our senses change—taste buds diminish. Most things don't taste like they used to. Smells may become more bothersome. Your eyes aren't so sharp. Pick out a nice pair of statement glasses and get on with it.

7. Hearing…What?
8. Migraines become less bothersome; that's good news.
9. Fear of falling is more common. That's because we're losing our sense of touch. If there is a handrail, hold on to it.
10. Our hair, eyebrows, and eyelashes are thinning.
11. Power naps become more frequent.
12. Belly fat increases. Oh yeah. It sure does.
13. Maybe you experience less stress. If only…
14. Facial hair—the hair on my husband's head found its way to my chin, while the hair on my head is disappearing along with my memory.
15. We complain A LOT!

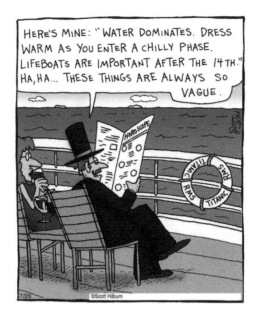

WHAT THE STARS SAY ABOUT YOU

AQUARIUS
January 20 - February 18

1. Humanitarian
2. Independent
3. Deep thinker
4. Aloof

PISCES
February 19 – March 20

1. Compassionate
2. Wise
3. Intuitive
4. Sometimes plays the victim

ARIES
March 21 - April 19

1. Competitive
2. Confident
3. Honest
4. Impulsive

TAURUS
April 20 – May 20

1. Stable
2. Devoted
3. Practical
4. Possessive

GEMINI
May 21 – June 20

1. Affectionate
2. Curious
3. Open minded
4. Inconsistent

CANCER
June 21- July 22

1. Loyal
2. Tenacious
3. Sympathetic
4. Moody

LEO
July 23 – August 22

1. Generous
2. Funny
3. Creative
4. Stubborn

VIRGO
August 23 – September 22

1. Kind
2. Loyal
3. Practical
4. Critical

LIBRA
September 23 – October 22

1. Social
2. Diplomatic
3. Gracious
4. Carries a grudge

SCORPIO
October 23 – November 21

1. Brave
2. Resourceful
3. A loyal friend
4. Distrusting

SAGITTARIUS
November 22 – December 21

1.   Good sense of humor
2.   Generous
3.   Curious
4.   Impatient

CAPRICORN
December 22 – January 19

1.   Self-controlled
2.   Responsible
3.   Traditional
4.   Condescending

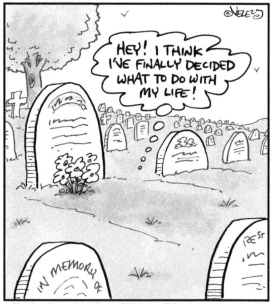

Fred raises the "Late Bloomer" bar to a new level.

LATE BLOOMERS
AND WE'RE NOT TALKING UNDERGARMENTS

These go-getters epitomize Over-Sixty: Shades of Brilliance:

- Grandma Moses – started painting at 76 years of age.
- James Parkinson – identified Parkinson's Disease at the age of 62.
- Frank McCourt – took up writing at 65. *Angela's Ashes* won the Pulitzer Prize and National Book Critics Circle Award.
- Colonel Sanders - started developing Kentucky Fried in his 60s.
- Peter Mark Roget – at the age of 73, published the first edition of Roget's Thesaurus.

- Benjamin Franklin – signed the Declaration of Independence at 70.
- Nelson Mandela – became president of South Africa at 76.
- Laura Ingalls Wilder – published her first book, *Little House on the Prairie*, at 65.
- Nola Ochs - was 95 when she became the oldest college graduate.
- Barbara Hillary – at 75, became one the oldest individuals to reach the North Pole.
- Daniel Defoe – wrote *Robinson Crusoe* at 60 years of age.
- Sir William Crookes - invented the first instruments to study radioactivity at age 68.

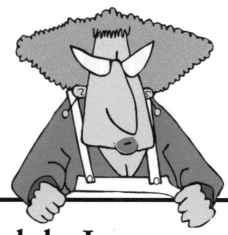

"I tried the Japanese method of decluttering where you hold every object that you own and if it does not bring you joy, you throw it away. So far I've thrown out all of my vegetables, my bra, my bills, the scale, a mirror and my treadmill."

—Author Unknown

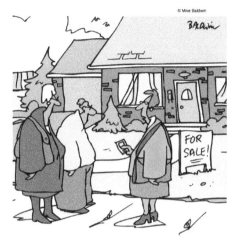

"Empty-nesters. They're hoping to sell before the flock tries to move back in."

DOWNSIZING YOUR HOME

If you think a large home is no longer easy to maintain, you may want to consider downsizing. This is the perfect time to start putting the wheels in motion because the first item on the list will probably be the most difficult.

- Get rid of the majority of your stuff. The boxes of items you never go into but saved "just in case." If you have bunches of books, sell them to second-hand stores or give them away. And if they're in bad condition, throw them away. Your eyesight is not going to get any sharper. And a tablet or e-Reader can not only hold a thousand books, but you can make the font larger and easier to read. Obviously, I'm not telling you to throw away your cherished collection of signed first editions. I'm telling you to sell them. Or give them to your children.

- Leave big bulky furniture behind. Sell it. Donate it. Give it to friends and family. Sure, you can take furniture with you, but if you have a heavy couch that seats seven people (like I do), keeping it is not downsizing. You'll probably have fewer rooms, and they may be smaller rooms. You'll suffocate, or bang your aging hips and knees, so get rid of bulky furniture now, so you don't have to pay to move it.

- When selecting new furniture, look for items that are easy to get out of and don't have sharp edges that can make your hips, knees, or toes black and blue when you bang into them.

There are considerations to keep in mind before you move into a smaller home. And if you have the time, you can make sure everything is done ahead of time.

- Get a grip. Lever handles are better than doorknobs.

- You're getting older. We're wishing you no harm, but you may want to make sure all interior doorways are wide enough to accommodate a future wheelchair. When you're 99, you'll thank us.

- Keep interior doorways simple. Don't use a door if you don't have to. Use a door that's easy to maneuver if you do, like a well-maintained pocket door. You don't want a door that swings into you if you use a wheelchair or walker.

- Avoid slippery floors. You may hate carpeting because it gets dirty quickly and is bad for allergies, but it's softer to fall on. Polished floors may be easier to clean but are slippery and could be the enemy of your hips. This is a 50-50 decision.

- Select a home that's light and bright. Our aging retinas don't see as well as they used to. Blame it on aging eye muscles and shrinking pupils. You'll want to make sure every room is well lit.

- Consider a bidet. Wiping your butt can be difficult when arthritis is acting up. Besides, you'll save on toilet paper.

- Many smaller homes may have combination tubs with showers. But you're not going to be able to climb into a tub forever. Look for walk-in showers that don't have a threshold, so you walk right into them without tripping. Use a shower bench if you need to sit down. A hand-held sprayer is good, too, so you can reach it while sitting. If you need to have a tub, consider one with a side panel door. And grab bars. Wet areas are slippery. Grab bars are a godsend.

- Having outdoor space is nice, but a large yard needs maintenance. You're downsizing. Unless you love mowing the lawn, planting flowers, or weeding the garden, you may also want to downsize your yard.

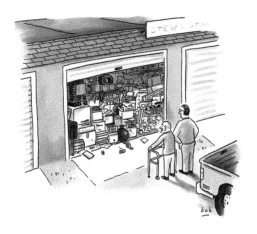

"One day Son all this will be yours."

DECLUTTERING YOUR HOUSE

- Start with simple goals—like today, I will throw ten things away. Or, today, I will just sort through the top drawer of the desk. Then do it.

- Study the item you no longer love. If it's in good condition, donate it. If it's chipped, torn, or broken, throw it away. If it's dirty, clean it, and then decide if it deserves space in your life.

- Declutter one room at a time. You'll be able to see results sooner than if you spread your work out all over your home.

- It's hard to get rid of things that mean a lot to us. If a tambourine reminds you of dancing on stage on your 18th birthday, take a picture and put it in a scrapbook. Then either give the item away or throw it away. Stuff can take up an entire room. A scrapbook can be kept in a single drawer.

- If you've either gained or lost weight and haven't worn something in the past couple of years, give it away before it goes completely out of style, so at least someone can get some use out of it.

- There are many ways to dispose of unwanted items: consignment shops, charitable organizations, a dumpster, eBay, or online sales venues. Just do it.

- Throwing unwanted clutter in a dumpster doesn't take much time. You won't make any money from it, but the reclaimed space you get back is priceless.

- If you're stuck on an item's value, you can always sell it. Selling items online takes time setting up an account, writing a description, and taking pictures. Then there's shipping, which can be a pain in the butt. But you will still gain space and maybe a few bucks.

- If your "clutter" is made up of small items that you need to hold on to, invest in decorative baskets. I like baskets with lids. When you're looking for small electronic adapters or phone chargers, it's easier when you know they're all in the same basket. And you'll never see the mess unless you need something.

- Every time you declutter, be it for one hour or one day, put aside a few dollars in an oversized mug or a drawer. By the time the room is done, you may be able to splurge on a can of paint to brighten up the space or a few new baskets for the next room.

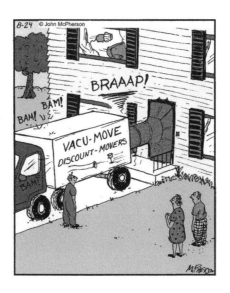

ME CASA? NEW CASA?

Thinking of moving? Want to be closer to your kids? Want to be as far away as possible from your kids?

Or perhaps you need a change of scenery. Whatever your reasons—planning a move is a huge undertaking, so talk to a professional.

According to the U.S. Census Bureau and SeniorScore™, here are some of the best states for 60 plussers in no particular order:

- Virginia—provides excellent health care, low taxes, and friendly people.
- Hawaii—is great for outdoor activities, property taxes are on the lower side, and it has good health care.
- South Carolina—has excellent weather, wonderful parks and beaches, and affordable living.

- North Carolina—has an affordable cost of living and lots of outdoor activities.
- Idaho—has beautiful national parks, is not too populated, and it's affordable. It also has lots of potatoes.
- Florida—need we say more? Fun, affordable living costs, great health care.
- Texas—excellent health care, good climate, affordable cost of living.
- Arizona—high senior population, easy on the pocketbook, tons of fun in the sun.
- West Virginia—checks all the boxes. Affordable living, quality health care, and low taxes.

According to SmartAsset.com, in 2018, nearly one million people, over sixty, moved across state lines.

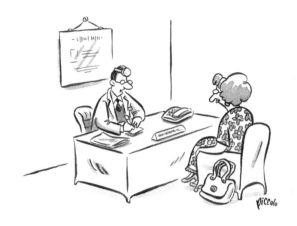

*"I'm going to prescribe medical marijuana
and sour cream & onion tortilla chips."*

SENIOR STONERS

Grandmas got the munchies, and I know why—so, throw away those painkillers and have a CBD gummy bear instead.

Remember the movie, *Starting Over with Jill Clayburgh?* There was a scene where she was having, if I remember correctly, a panic attack. She was lying on a bed in Bloomingdales hysterical, and a guy screamed, "Does anyone have a Valium?" Everyone opened up their pocketbooks and reached in. A very funny moment. And at that time, very hush-hush. Today it's a totally different story.

• Marijuana has increased by 71% in adults 50 and over—that's according to a New York University Study. And according to the *Journal of the American Medical Association*, "the numbers of American seniors over 65 who now smoke marijuana or use edible versions increased two-fold between 2015-2018. Reasons could be that the older generation is familiar with pot because of their past use, plus it's more available.

- Dispensaries can now be found in many states. They offer everything from medical marijuana and edibles to instruction on its uses. All you have to do is look online for one near you.
- I had a friend who ate brownies laced with pot every night because of his insomnia. "I slept like a baby," he said. And he woke up feeling alert. He always told me to "try this," placing a brownie under my nose. It looked so good, but I declined. Too many calories. He was one of the older folks that used weed to treat his diseases and ease his symptoms.
- There are topicals as well to ameliorate pain. CBD oil or pills without the high ingredient THC is also available. I used to give CBD oil to my dog, Bentley. He had diabetes.
- I read that people are having pot parties, much like the Tupperware parties we had years ago. They hire someone in the business to educate them about what cannabis is, its many uses and offer baking recipes.
- If you are so inclined to add pot as an ingredient, you might want to try: www.solisbetter.com, www.marijuanamommy.com, www.cannabischeri.com, etc.
- There are many drawbacks. If you have pre-existing conditions such as heart problems or diabetes or you're on certain medications, it's best to check with your doctor before using cannabis because of contra-indications. Keep in mind that experts say marijuana has become more potent over the years and could cause problems in an aging body.

There are side effects. Short-term ones may include:

- Deficiencies in memory

- Difficulties in comprehension or learning
- Increased heart rate
- Anxiety

And long-term effects could include:

- Memory loss
- Judgment impairment
- Respiratory problems
- Addiction

On the plus side, MedicalNewsToday.com says marijuana may relieve certain kinds of pain, reduce nausea, and ease some side effects of chemotherapy.

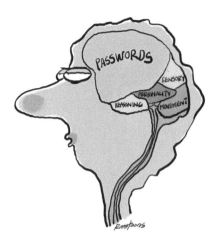

WHAT TO DO IF YOUR PASSWORDS ARE COMPROMISED

It was the dawn of a new day. My morning routine was underway until I sat down at the computer and waited for it to load.

OMG! Notice after notice. Some of my passwords, 91 of them, have been compromised. Are you kidding me? Do you have any idea how many websites have my credit card?

First things first:

- Try not to panic, which is exactly what I did.
- Take a deep breath. Try to keep your blood pressure under stroke level.
- Run a virus and malware scan.
- Google *What does it mean if my passwords were compromised?* And *What should I do?* When you see all the sites and all the

159

links provided, take another deep breath, and try not to shake.
- When all the information starts unfolding, and you still don't know what to do, walk away from the computer. Take a break.
- Now sit down and face the task at hand. A safe bet is to get out a piece of paper, make a list of all your new passwords, and put it in a drawer or someplace accessible.
- Utilize password manager apps, but remember they, too, are on the cloud.
- If you need to change your passwords, it's best to make them long using letters, symbols, and numbers.
- Enable security settings, for example, two-factor authentication.
- Don't use the same password twice. Each website should have a unique password.
- Keep your computer updated.
- And if you have a computer consultant, scream *Help!*

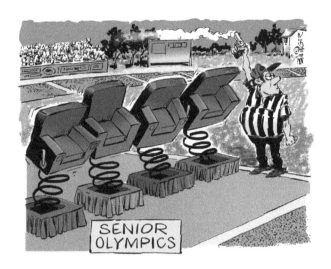

REGULAR PEOPLE DOING AMAZING THINGS AFTER 60

- Gladys Burrill – ran and completed a marathon at 92 and earned her place in the *Guinness Book of World Records* for being the oldest female to do so.
- Teiichi Igarashi – climbed Mt. Fuji at 100 years old and had been climbing the mountain since he was 89.
- Diana Nyad – was the first person to swim 53 straight hours and 110 miles from Cuba to Florida at 64 years old.
- William Ivy Baldwin – at 82, walked across a canyon on a tightrope.
- Momofuku Ando – invented the Ramen Cup Noodles at 61 (and college students around the world are thankful).
- Oscar Swahn – competed and earned a medal in the 1920 Summer Olympics at 72.

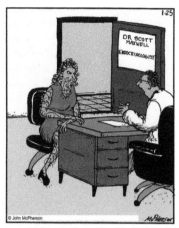

"Before we discuss the side effects, Mrs. Gimler, I need to know if the hormone therapy is helping your mood."

WHY THE OLD WHORE MOANED

- She lost her sense of taste.

- Her belly, butt, and boobs all sagged.

- Her nose began to drip at will.

- Cracked and brittle nails.

- Loss of short-term memory and long-term's not so good.

- Body odor changes.

- Her farts were no longer under her control.

- Two words: bad knees.

- A new pain every day.

- Dry eye, dry skin, dry vagina.

- "I'm shrinking!"

- Thinning skin bruises easily.

- Thinning hair, except on her chin, in her nose, and coming out of her ears.

- Body weight redistribution.

- She couldn't read the fine print. Or the regular print. And the large print was fuzzy.

- Two more words: urinary incontinence.

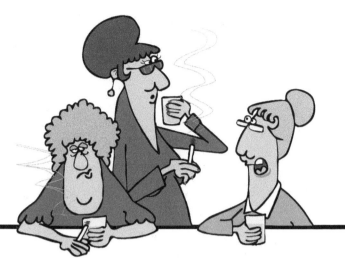

"You know you've reached middle age when you're told to slow down by your doctor, instead of by the police."

—Joan Rivers

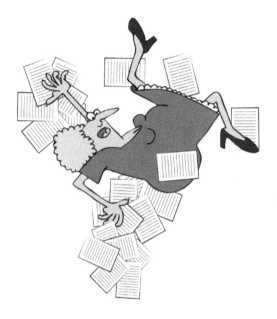

Productivity

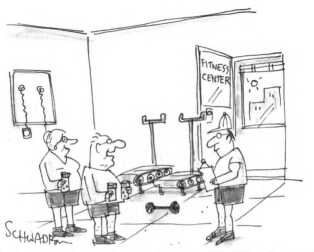

"WE'D JUST LIKE TO GET IN SHAPE TO OPEN OUR MEDICATION BOTTLES."

YOU'RE RETIRED. NOW WHAT?

- Take that college course you always wanted to take. Many colleges and universities offer online degrees. You can either take classes in the comfort of your home or mingle with others in a classroom.
- Join a book club. Your first choice of books should be *Over-Sixty: Shades of Gray*. Just saying…
- Go to lectures. Many Y's, assisted living facilities, libraries, and towns have programs and guest speakers.
- Join a club or class, whether it be walking, art, current events, exercise, etc.
- Volunteer.
- Make yourself available to help out your neighbors and friends.
- Take the time to do what you've always wanted to do but never got around to doing.

- Maybe start a small business that caters to seniors' needs: transportation services, companions for hire, home services like cleaning, food shopping, etc.
- If you have the expertise or a degree, be it in history, art, or physical movement, teach a small group in a place like a Y, library, or senior center.
- Create a small business, house sitting, pet sitting, or plant watering. Even taking in the mail when people go on vacation.
- Learn a new skill.
- Look for freelance or temp work.

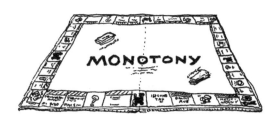

S. McC

TWELVE WAYS TO FIGHT BOREDOM

1. Clean your house, attic, basement, or garage. Give away the stuff you've been meaning to get rid of for years. (We never said these are *fun* ways not to be bored).
2. Clean up your emails, followed by the rest of the files on your computer.
3. Give yourself a spa day—wash your hair, polish your nails, and relax with a facial.
4. There's always television.
5. Play board games like scrabble. Or play it on your computer or tablet if there's no one handy to play against.
6. Put together your own list of how not to be bored tomorrow.
7. Put together a gratitude list.
8. Now is the time to apologize for past events or situations that made you feel uncomfortable.
9. Write a letter in longhand to an old friend.

10. Listen to nostalgic music and remember the good times.
11. Bake a cake, cookies, bread, or a pie. If you're dieting, find creative ways to cut calories/carbs /fats without sacrificing flavor.
12. Plant a garden or some flower beds.

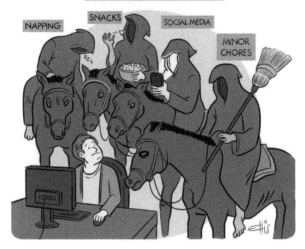

PROCRASTINATION PARALYSIS

"My mother always told me I wouldn't amount to anything because I procrastinate. I said, 'Just wait.'" —Judy Tenuta

When it comes to procrastinating, there are several reasons why we may put things off:

- Self-doubt—feeling inadequate that you can't accomplish the task successfully
- Anxiety
- Bad mood
- Insecurity
- The importance of the task at hand
- Thinking the job will take too long
- Too many external stimuli

- You just don't want to do it
- Lack of motivation

Experts say 20% of individuals identify as procrastinators, and men procrastinate more than women. You don't have to convince me! According to a survey on the subject, 94% of the responses said procrastination has a "negative effect on their happiness."

For argument's sake, let's call procrastination *taking a break*. It can have benefits:

- It can rest your mind and reduce your stress level.
- It can unclutter the clutter.
- It could make room for creativity. After all, coffee isn't the only thing that needs to percolate.

Now, let's talk about solutions:

- Set goals.
- Create a to-do list—don't overburden your list with to-dos.
- Try to manage your emotions.
- Try not to think about being "perfect."
- Create realistic time management techniques.
- Reward yourself.
- Make your surroundings comfortable, so you enjoy being there.
- Remember how good you felt when you finished the last project.

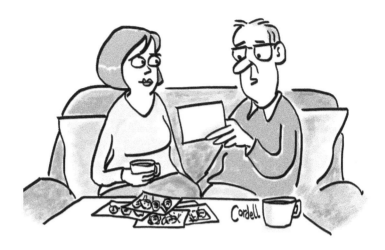

"Didn't we look young when we were young."

PICTURE THIS

How many old photographs have you collected over the years?

In my home, from generation to generation, they've been hanging around in boxes, in albums, and on the walls. And to top it off, I don't know a majority of these people. I inherited a shitload of photos from my mother after she died. And the last thing I want to do is dump them on my daughter.

Time to divest. The thought—daunting! However, this pain-in-the-ass project can begin this way:

- Organize your thoughts. Figure out how you will approach the project.

- Begin by doing what's easiest for you. Step by step. Box by box. Try not to think you'll never finish.
- As you review your photos, toss out those that are damaged, blurred, or torn…you get the idea.
- What makes it challenging and more time-consuming is getting lost in nostalgia. Try to avoid lingering.
- Separate and classify the photos into three groups: keep, toss, and who are these people?
- I asked my daughter if she wanted any of the pictures I saved. We made another pile. We also walked around the house to see if there was anything else she wanted, like heirlooms, dishes, her baby toys, anything and everything else. My Last Will & Testament will be shorter, my home emptier.
- If friends and relatives have admired something in your home and it's on your get-this-out-of-here list, offer it to them.
- As a matter of fact, have a party.

"Always be nice to your children because they are the ones who will choose your rest home."

—Phyllis Diller

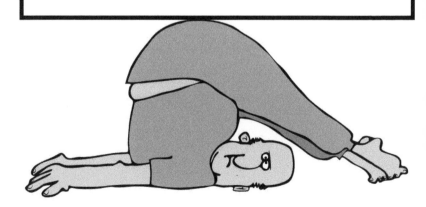

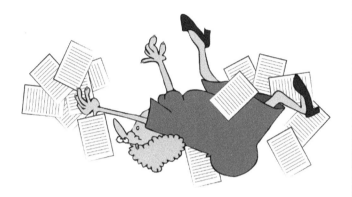

Relationships

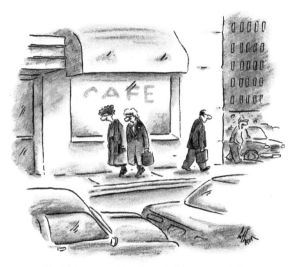

"I'm having my wedding ring melted down into a bullet."

I DO. I DID. I'M DONE. RELATIONSHIP DEAL BREAKERS

Trying to end a relationship with your partner, friend, or anyone in your life that is causing you more angst than joy is never easy. You might say to yourself, "Well, just like a pimple on my ass, I'll get used to it," just to avoid the discomfort of breaking up. But why should you?

Here are some red flags to alert you as to whether you should pursue a relationship or, if you're already in one, how to end it:

- You start feeling uneasy with the thought of being with them. So, you make up excuses to avoid them.
- Beware of new acquaintances who share too much personal information right off the bat. Boy! I could write a book about this experience.
- They make you doubt yourself.

- They put you down, often in front of other people, and then say, "I'm only joking."
- They monopolize the conversation and talk mainly about themselves. They hardly show interest in you or gossip about other people. And for sure, if they're gossiping about people, they're also talking behind your back.
- They ask for favors more than they're willing to give of themselves. It's a take me, buy me, show me, do for me—with no return.
- They're rude to other people.
- Apologizing doesn't exist.
- They're unsupportive.
- They exhibit physical and emotional abuse.
- Often, they're reluctant to be with your friends.
- They're possessive.
- They overstep boundaries.
- They're moody.

Now, you have to put the pedal to the metal, drive forward and treat yourself to some self-care. Neil Sedaka's song said it best, "Breaking Up is Hard to Do."

- Depending upon the reason for the breakup, you will feel better about yourself if you are respectful and honest.
- Speak with someone you trust beforehand to better prepare yourself. Bounce ideas around. Know what you are going to say.
- You may want to mention that your life is taking a different direction. Relationships don't have to be toxic to want to move on. People outgrow people.
- Prepare yourself for reactions.
- Don't underestimate your gut.
- Don't hang on to the thoughts and feelings of breaking up. Do it.

- Try meeting face to face; it's most respectful. Don't text or email.
- You can make yourself unavailable, but that just prolongs the agony.
- Say nothing on social media.

If they ask why you're splitting, tell them. Give them a chance to respond. Be kind.

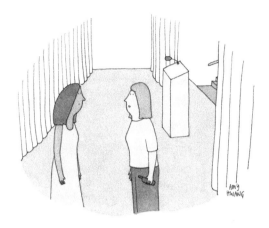

"If you're nervous, just imagine everyone in the audience without their Spanx."

HOW TO MAKE YOUR MARK WITHOUT A SHARPIE

- Know your audience.
- Be yourself.
- Smile.
- Be punctual.
- Engage with others; be attentive.
- Have a positive disposition.
- Wear confidence.
- Dress according to the occasion.
- If you have a sense of humor, use it, but don't overtake the conversation.
- Be honest; save the BS.
- Make people feel important, and ask them questions about themselves.
- And like they say, "honesty is the best policy."

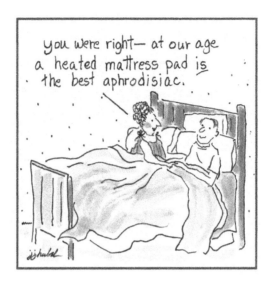

APHRODISIACS

- Artichokes
- Asparagus (a popular aphrodisiac but also considered a turnoff because it makes your pee smell bad)
- Avocados
- Bananas (it's not the shape; it's the potassium)
- Chocolate
- Fenugreek (a manly herb)
- Figs
- Ginkgo
- Ginseng
- Maca (said to increase libido and reduce erectile dysfunction)
- Oysters
- Pistachio nuts
- Pomegranates
- Pumpkin seeds

- Red wine
- Saffron
- Salmon
- Saw palmetto (reportedly improves prostate health)
- Spicy chili peppers (are there unspicy ones?)
- Spinach (it worked for Popeye)
- Strawberries
- Tribulus (another manly herb)
- Watermelon
- A sexy partner who turns you on.

You may want to check with your doctor before using any of the listed herbs or supplements because they could interfere with the medications you may be taking.

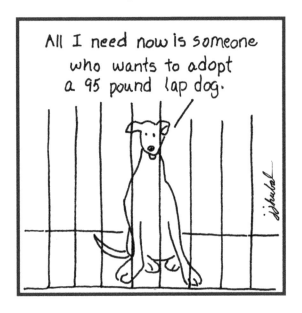

All I need now is someone who wants to adopt a 95 pound lap dog.

SENIORS HELPING SENIORS

Yes, I am a dog lover. I'm an animal lover. But if I brought home a pigmy goat or a pot-belly pig, my husband would have a canary. I like birds too! I have rescued many dogs. And why not? It makes my home complete. It makes me feel good that I saved a life.

Long story short, dogs became domesticated from wolves thousands of years ago when they wandered into the campsites of hunters looking for food. After a while, they started protecting those sites, becoming buddies of these hunters. Hence, our best friends. They have always been there for us. So, we need to show up for them.

Way too many shelters euthanize older animals to make room for the very popular puppy. I know it's hard to resist a puppy. But keep in mind that the older dog comes with many benefits like house training, for one, and they are just as loving, maybe more

182

so, because they know they've been rescued. You have essentially become their hero. You may not know their history, but with proper training and love, you will create your own history.

Two years ago, I rescued Coco, a nine-year-old mixed breed. I was specifically looking for a senior because, like us folk, we are overlooked, cast aside, and ignored when we reach a certain age.

We will grow older together and stay healthier because:

- Having a pet lowers your blood pressure.
- It reduces stress and pushes you to exercise by walking them.
- You never feel alone.
- They provide companionship.
- They can help improve your social life. So many people stop people walking a dog. It starts with a conversation, and hey, you never know.
- They add structure to your day; you must walk and feed them at certain times.
- Some dogs can even detect illness.
- When I feel overwhelmed, I hug Coco, and I feel calmer.
- According to the American Kennel Club, dogs help seniors with "cognitive function and social interaction."
- It feels so good to experience an uncomplicated love.

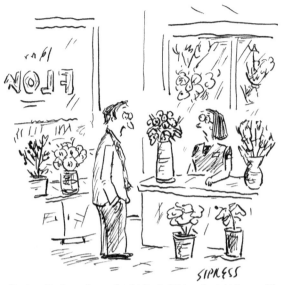

"I need something that says, 'I'm sorry about that thing I said that caused you to totally overreact.'"

YOU'RE PISSED, NOW WHAT?

Winning an argument may not be as important as losing a relationship. So…

- Take a deep breath and try to stay calm. Challenging, I know.
- Focus. Don't go off on tangents. Too often, when we hold stuff in, we're all over the place.
- Listen. Let the other person finish what they're saying.
- Asking questions about how, what, and why they feel a certain way is an opportunity for deeper communication and understanding.
- When they are making a stronger point than yours, say so, and give them credit for it. Maybe you'll be able to see where they are coming from and gain another perspective.

184

- Losing often can be a win. Sometimes you have to change your mindset.
- Don't be afraid to talk to the person just because you may not like the consequences. If you let stuff bottle up, you will explode! Trust me on this.
- Yes, honesty is the best policy, but cushion your remarks. Be tactful. Be respectful.
- Make sure the points you are trying to make are accurate.

If you can accomplish any of these tips, you will have walked away a winner.

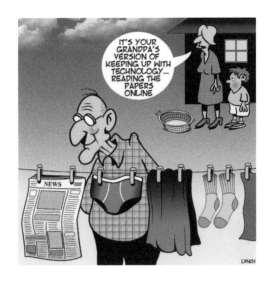

THERE'S NOTHING LIKE BEING A GRANDPARENT

My friends who are grandparents have always said, having a grandchild is beyond their wildest expectations. It is "Amazing!" Of this, I am sure.

There seem to be lots of senior grandparents, 83% according to the Pew Research Center, who say being a grandparent is the best thing about getting older.

We've spoken to some grannies and pop-pops, and they had plenty to say.

Nana Ann:

♥ Watching them grow! Observing their development, delighting in every new mastery from their first smile to their first words to their teaching ME how to use Instagram. I am on the journey without the heavy lifting!

♥ Introducing them to new ideas and activities. Spending leisure time without the worries and responsibilities. I can actually be present and available to share in their experiences.
♥ Watching my daughter being a mother. I am in awe that MY little girl is now a woman who raises her children with so much love and wisdom.
♥ The biggest challenge is to always keep in mind that I am the NANA, not the parent.

Grandma Joan:

♥ Whether they want me to buy them something or take them somewhere, I always respond by saying, "If mom and dad say it's all right."
♥ I also try to instill in them some semblance of not being takers.
♥ Being a grandparent doesn't come with the anxiety we had when raising our own kids.

Mimi Brenda:

♥ It's hard to believe that my kids have kids. It's almost as though you love them more because you don't have the responsibility and guilt of raising them. It's a wonderful thing.
♥ As far as boundaries are concerned, if I take them somewhere, it is understood that I have carte blanche to buy them things.
♥ If you have a good relationship with your children, you'll have a good relationship with your grandchildren.

Poppy Don:

♥ The joy for me is knowing I'm making my grandkids happy and being involved in their lives. It's wonderful watching them grow.

Grandpa Don G:

♥ I love being with my grandkids because it's like watching myself grow up.

Papa Steve & Grammy Cindy:

♥ Being able to contribute to another child's growth and development as one watches them go from infancy to adulthood.
♥ Experiencing your grandchild's growth over the years and having great pride in their accomplishments.
♥ Having your grandchild share their successes.
♥ Special feelings of love from your grandchild, no matter their age.

These are the challenges grandparents say they face:

♥ Trying not to spoil them excessively.
♥ Not criticizing or judging.
♥ Finding special activities, such as songs, games, or events that will create memories.
♥ Trying to include both parents when issues arise.
♥ Respecting your child's decision.

Because as one grandparent said anonymously:

"They go back to their parents."

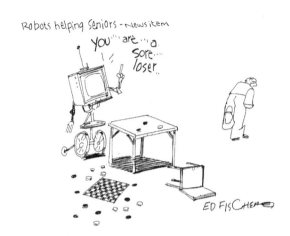

TEAMWORK!

This list is geared toward *younger* older adults who can help *older* seniors with daily tasks. On the upside, it could turn into a small business with flexible hours, petty cash if you choose to charge, and it could provide you with feelings of productivity after retirement. You could:

- Help someone look for a home health aide to assist them with personal hygiene, medications, etc.
- Provide transportation to appointments.
- Provide home services like cleaning, shopping, or cooking.
- Companionship. Some seniors just need someone to talk to, to read to them, have afternoon tea with, or perhaps a game of gin rummy.

If you have the experience and knowledge in a specialized field, you could also:

- Help someone with medical claims
- Provide nutrition counseling
- Train individuals how to exercise properly
- Retrofit seniors' homes to accommodate wheelchairs or install safety features like grab bars

As the old commercial said: *Reach out and touch someone.*

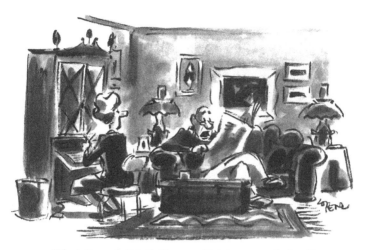

"Why don't we make it simple this year, and just give everyone the finger?"

FIVE TIPS TO GET YOU THROUGH THE HOLIDAYS

Unrealistic expectations, combined with too little time, too much pressure, and financial concerns, may all contribute to stress during the holidays. You've probably heard the song, "It's the most wonderful time of the year." And almost everyone has heard the saying, "Bah, humbug!"

Here are five tips to help you keep the holidays in perspective:

1. It doesn't hurt to say, "Happy Holidays!"
2. Don't be afraid to say, "No."
3. Go ahead, eat a piece of chocolate. It will make you feel good. (Darker is better).
4. Toast the New Year with your favorite beverage, even if it's Boost or Ensure.
5. Breathe.

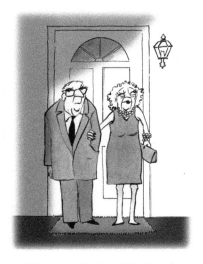

All dressed up without the slightest idea why.

WHEN YOUR BACK GOES OUT MORE OFTEN THAN YOU DO

Looking for a not-too-strenuous activity for a fun date? Try:

Lectures
Art Classes
Book Clubs
Films
Art Galleries
Museums
Wine tastings
Picnics
Double dating
Miniature golf
Dinner cruises
Afternoon tea

Concerts
Country fairs
Watching the sunset
Going out for ice cream
Going "parking"
Seeing a Broadway-style show or play
Visiting a carnival
Spending a day at the beach
Berry picking
Eating pancakes for dinner
Visiting a farmer's market
Karaoke
Ballroom dancing
Planetariums

While there are a lot of other wonderful activities like hiking, roller skating, and bowling, they might be better left for younger people with better healing powers. Nothing says "AKK," like a bad back.

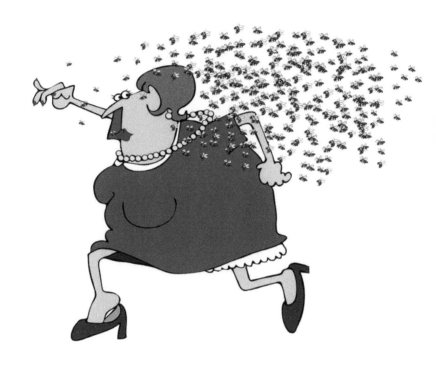

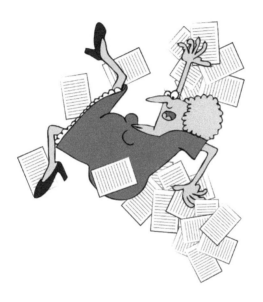

Safety

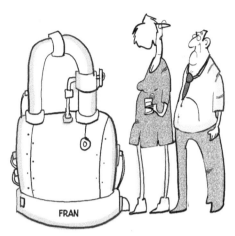

WELL, I'M NOT SURE WHAT IT IS, BUT IT WAS 50% OFF IN
THE SALE SO I THOUGHT I'D GET ONE BEFORE THEY SOLD OUT!

NINE NIFTY GADGETS & GIZMOS

1. Grabber tool for grabbing things on a high shelf or that have fallen on the floor.
2. Portable suction grab bar that you can move from room to room.
3. Extra-long shoehorn because bending over just ain't what it used to be.
4. Pocket magnifier for the small print, which at our age, is usually the whole page.
5. Compression socks if you want to avoid deep vein thrombosis.
6. Motion sensor light to brighten what's ahead.
7. Digital thermometer, so every time someone asks, "Do you have a fever?" you'll know the answer.
8. Toilet seat bidet just in case another pandemic results in another toilet paper shortage.
9. Caption Phone (provided free by the government) prints out a conversation in easy-to-read text.

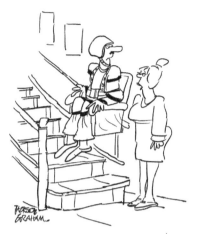

"FOR GOODNESS SAKE EDGAR – IT'S A
STAIR LIFT NOT A MOON ROCKET!"

TWENTY-TWO TERRIFIC TIPS FOR AGING IN PLACE

1. Install grab bars in showers and baths.
2. Use a transfer bench for baths.
3. Have a shower chair handy.
4. Use non-slip strips in bathtubs and showers.
5. Consider using a toilet frame, turning your bathroom bowl into a throne!
6. Install night lights and motion sensor lighting.
7. Consider a stair lift.
8. Remove rugs that could be a trip hazard.
9. Have a fire extinguisher on hand (most fires start in the kitchen, so that's a good place to keep one).
10. Put together or buy a first aid kit.
11. Remove unnecessary clutter.
12. Wear secure footwear.
13. Don't go barefoot (don't expect Carol to follow this rule because she feels more secure feeling the floor under her feet for now).

14. Empty lint from clothes dryers to avoid fires.
15. Go slow. After all, what's your hurry?
16. Try to live on one level (your knees will thank you, and there are no stairs to fall down).
17. Install smoke and carbon monoxide detectors if you don't already have them, and check them annually.
18. Create an exit plan for all areas of your home.
19. Place a contact list in an easy-to-find spot with information about family and doctors to call in an emergency.
20. Consider wearing a medical alert button (it requires a monthly subscription).
21. Switch to a cane with a multi-prong bottom for greater stability.
22. If you hate using a cane or walker but feel unsteady on your feet, think like a cruise ship designer, and put handrails along the walls. They'll make you more stable while helping you get where you want to go.

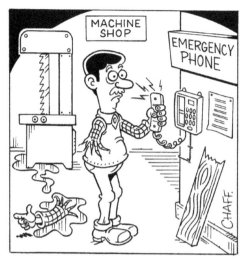

"...PRESS 1 TO BOOK AN APPOINTMENT...PRESS 2 FOR A DOCTOR...PRESS 3 FOR AN AMBULANCE..."

MUST HAVES FOR YOUR FIRST AID KIT

- Assorted size bandages
- Assorted size sterile gauze pads
- Antibiotic ointment
- Alcohol cleansing pads
- Antiseptic wipes
- Antiseptic ointment
- Adhesive cloth tape
- Ice pack
- Non-latex gloves
- Acetaminophen or ibuprofen
- Oral thermometer
- Small scissors
- Tweezer
- Elastic wrap (like an Ace Bandage)
- CPR mask

- Calamine lotion
- Moldable splints
- Instant cold packs for injuries
- First aid manual
- Tourniquet

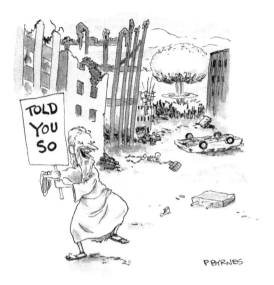

WHAT TO PACK IN A DISASTER PREPAREDNESS KIT

These items will not sustain you through an apocalypse, but they could help if you're temporarily forced to deal with the immediate effects of a hurricane or fire or if you need to flee your home in a hurry when you need to get the hell out of Dodge.

- Three days of non-perishable food items and water
- Medications
- Cash
- Flashlight
- Batteries
- Hand-crank or battery-powered radio
- Copies of birth certificates, passports, insurance cards, and other important documents
- Can opener
- Disposable utensils and plates

- Pet food and meds if you have an animal
- Back up cell phone battery or solar charger
- Change of clothes
- Personal toiletries like a toothbrush and comb
- Multi-tool or Swiss Army knife
- First Aid kit
- Candles
- Waterproof matches or lighter
- Wet wipes
- N95 masks
- Latex gloves
- Blankets
- And alcohol (not the kind you drink)

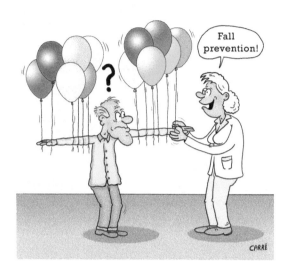

PREVENTING FALLS

An oft-quoted line from a commercial for a personal medical alert system that younger people joke about and older people fear is, "I've fallen, and I can't get up."

According to the National Institute of Aging, one in three people over the age of 65 falls each year. We can blame falls on any number of reasons:

- Eyesight
- Hearing
- Reflexes
- Medications
- Diseases like diabetes or heart disease
- Foot problems
- Muscle weakness

- Balance problems
- A rapid drop in blood pressure
- Confusion
- Trip hazards
- Wet floors
- Rushing

Prevention Tips:

- Stay physically active to maintain flexible joints and ligaments
- Get enough sleep
- Limit alcohol
- Use a cane or walker if you feel shaky
- Reduce trip hazards like loose rugs or objects on the floor (shopping bags, small boxes, decorative objects, books, clothing, etc.)
- Keep a flashlight by your bed at night to light your path
- Get up slowly to avoid a drop in blood pressure
- Be careful walking on snow and ice
- Wear non-skid, rubber-soled, low heel shoes
- Use night lights
- Arrange furniture, so it's not in your way
- Don't stand on a chair or ottoman to reach something high (Uh oh…)
- Know where your pets are

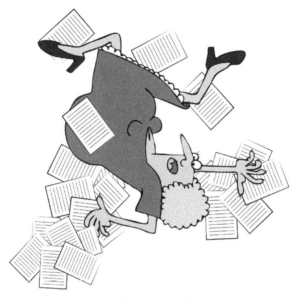

Self

Awareness

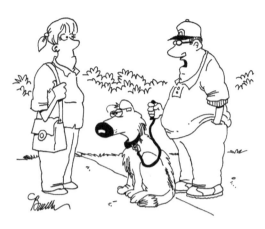

" I really didn't want him, but I need him to cover up the fact that I sometimes smell like a wet dog."

I SMELL OLD

My grandmother was an amazing woman. Unedited, very funny, and quite the fashionista. When she walked down the aisle at my wedding, it was my Nanny May who got the oohs and ahs. Young in spirit and young at heart, as they say.

However, when she reached a certain age, some age-related changes became more noticeable. She was shorter, and her mental capacity wasn't as sharp. But the most obvious difference was the way she smelled. The delicious fragrance of Chanel #5 that had once wrapped around her was replaced by a unique odor that I was unfamiliar with. Her hygiene was impeccable, so it wasn't that.

How does this happen?

1. Hormones. Sound familiar? As we age, the substances in our body change, producing a compound called Nonenal.
2. According to experts, Nonenal, is a chemical compound with

an unpleasant musty, grassy, or greasy odor.

3. The sweat glands (comprised of water and organic substances) produce what we know as our garden variety BO.

4. The sebaceous glands produce fatty acids, and when it doesn't oxidize, it releases a unique body odor. So, all the smelly stuff can become offensive.

5. It has nothing to do with cleanliness. No matter how much you scrub, you're kind of stuck with the stink.

6. It lingers on fabrics like clothes and bedding.

7. Stress can worsen the odor.

8. Did you know that middle-aged men, according to research, were the most stinky of the lot, while middle-aged women smelled the best? I missed my smell-good years.

I sometimes think I smell old. The scent of my grandmother still lingers on, which makes me self-conscious. I have often asked my daughter, "Do I smell old?" So far, so good.

What can we do?

9. It's quite natural to become immune to our own scent. So, smell your clothes, like your shirt collars and pillows. If they stink, well, then you know. I always smell my pillows, and to tell you the truth, not so good. So, into the washing machine they go.

10. Use purifying body washes, soaps with Persimmon extract or tannin, and Japanese Green Tea. It neutralizes the odor.

11. Persimmons have potent antiseptic properties. Google Persimmon or Japanese Persimmon soaps to locate a provider near you.

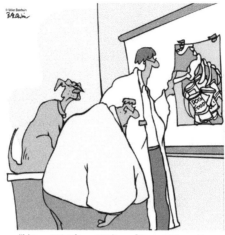

"He ... won't ... wait ... for ... me ... to ...
open ... the ...can."

WHY AM I MOVING SO SLOWLY?

It's not your imagination. It's not relativity (sorry, Einstein). It's simply that the changes in our bodies are working against us.

Here's the deal:

- As we age, muscle mass shrinks (3% or more a year).

- It can make it more challenging to recover from an injury.

- Muscle loss can mean the loss of independence.

- Lost muscle is usually replaced by fat.

- People lose more fast-twitch fibers (think: energy bursts), which results in becoming slower.

- We also lose slow-twitch fibers, but at a lesser rate, which weakens our endurance.

- Weak muscles make it harder to balance, which could result in falls.

- Strength training can slow down muscle loss and could reverse it.

When I was a teenager, I was on my high school track team. Hard to believe, but true. And I could really hold my own in the 25-yard dash. But nothing else. I couldn't win any race that required endurance. I think it's because I was probably born with more fast-twitch muscle fibers. And now they're dead.

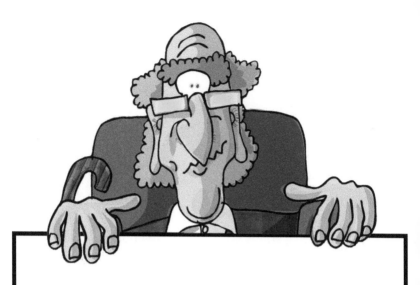

"People ask me what I'd most appreciate getting for my eighty-seventh birthday. I tell them, a paternity suit."

—George Burns

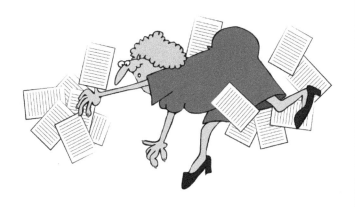

Sex After
Sixty

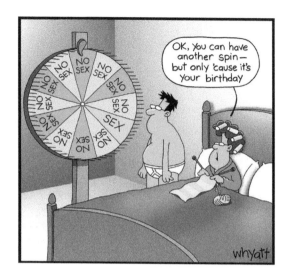

REASONS WHY YOU'VE LOST THAT LOVING FEELING

- Decreased libido (nothing going on down there)
- Dryness
- Painful penetration
- Difficulty in reaching a climax
- Relationship problems
- Physiological/psychological issues
- Medication
- Just plain tired or busy
- Not in the mood
- Reduced hormones
- You just don't like who you're with

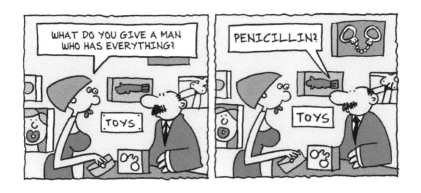

SEX TOYS

- Dildos. The size, of course, is up to you.
- Vibrators. There are hundreds to choose from. Go on-line and Google sex toys.
- Vibrating panties.
- Blow-up sex dolls.
- There are also gay sex toys, oral sex toys, men's sex toys. I'm telling you, for every hole and erogenous zone there is a sex toy.

Go to porn shops. They happen to be fun. Their contemporary cards are hysterical.

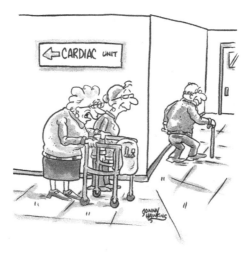

"We met in the ICU. We had a rheumatic encounter."

TEN WAYS TO RE-IGNITE PASSION

1. Exercise.
2. Quit smoking to improve blood flow.
3. Talk with your doctor about low-dose estrogen therapy.
4. Limit alcohol consumption. Too much liquor can inhibit sexual responses.
5. Control your weight. A healthy diet improves your stamina and body image perception.
6. Talk to your doctor.
7. Talk to your partner, tell them what you like.
8. Try new things. Be inventive.
9. Watch sultry movies together.
10. Remember: your body might have changed, but so has your partners.

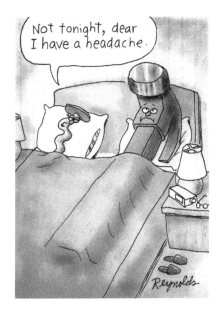

AVOIDING SEX WITHOUT OFFENDING YOUR PARTNER

Sex can be a schlepp, so how do you explain why it's just not working for you at the moment? These are the excuses I have used in the past:

- I'm too tired.
- I have a yeast infection.
- I have a UTI.
- Whatever physical ailment works (sinus infection, lower back pain, etc).
- I could say I had my period, but that has been *loooong* gone.

215

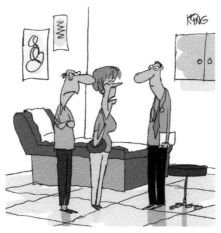

"My husband has lost his sex drive. What can we do to keep it that way?"

WOMANSPLAINING...

Here are some ways to keep your partner's feelings from being hurt when you don't feel like engaging in sex, so they won't take it personally and feel rejected (for a change):

1. Explain why you are saying no. If you are feeling stressed or have other emotional stuff getting in the way, share that.
2. Suggest another time. Sooner rather than later. Make a date.
3. Try other ways to connect: snuggling is always nice, a glass of wine, and good conversation.
4. Make it the idea of feeling close that's important. Sex doesn't have to be the end goal. (This obviously wasn't written by a man.)

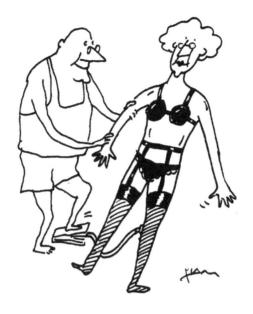

SIX WAYS TO SATISFY YOURSELF SEXUALLY

1. Masturbate. Trust me, you won't go blind! Learning about your body at any age is a good thing.
2. Watch porn. It's a turn-on. I can give you some titles.
3. Fantasize. Don't be afraid to go to places that might be unsettling. Remember, they are your fantasies. They are private. It's all in your head.
4. Read erotic stories. I remember I read The Story of O in college, and oh my god!
5. Check out audiobooks.com if you like sexy sounds.
6. Go to the Museum of Sex in NYC. It's not just toys.

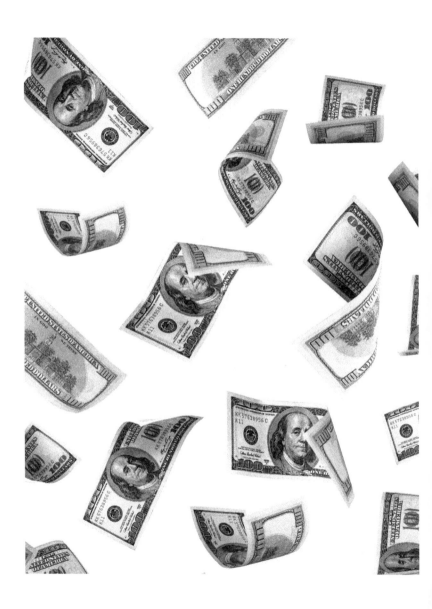

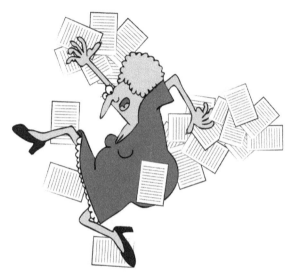

Show Me
the Money

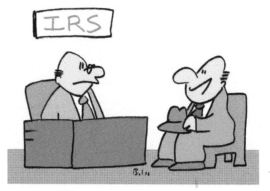

"Those 'reverse mortgage'
commercials got me to thinking —
Is there such a thing as reverse *taxes?*"

REVERSE MORTGAGE PROS & CONS

If you're over 62, own your home, and find yourself in a financial crunch, you may want to consider a reverse mortgage, which uses the equity in your home to help cover expenses. And if you're pissed off at your kids, it's a great way to keep them from inheriting your house. This article specifically addresses Home Equity Conversion Mortgages (HECMs).

Use a HECM to pay for such things as:

- Prescription drugs
- Home repairs
- Credit card debt
- Adult daycare
- Aging in place modifications

However, you should do your due diligence and learn what you're getting into.

Eligibility:

- All homeowners must be 62 or older.
- You must own the property outright or have paid down the mortgage by at least 80%.
- You must occupy the property as your primary residence.
- You cannot be delinquent on any federal debt.
- You must attend HUD counseling first.

Benefits:

- Home Equity Conversion Mortgages are regulated by the US Department of Housing and Urban Development (HUD) and the Federal Housing Administration (FHA).
- If you're over 62, you can get a "non-recourse loan," which means your children won't have to pay it back.
- There are no monthly payments for the homeowner(s).
- It's tax-free.
- It doesn't affect Social Security or Medicare benefits.
- No payments are due until the last living homeowner either moves away or dies.

Caveats:

- Payments can affect eligibility for Medicaid and similar needs-based programs. Medicaid eligibility varies from state to state, so you may want to consult an expert first.
- Homeowner(s) must keep homeowner's insurance and property tax payments up to date, as well as any Homeowner Association fees.

- Homeowner(s) must be committed to living in the home long-term.
- After all eligible homeowners permanently move away or pass on, the estate has 30 days to sell the home for fair market value, with the proceeds going to satisfy the loan.
- If your children or grandchildren anticipate inheriting your home, won't they be surprised!
- There are a lot of home equity loans on the market, but they don't necessarily have the benefits of a HECM. Choose wisely.

Costs:

- Like any mortgage, closing costs and fees (title search, appraisal, recording fees, etc.) must be paid upfront (but can be paid out of the proceeds).
- Mortgage Insurance Premiums (can be financed as part of the loan).
- Origination Fee – to compensate lenders for processing loans.
- Servicing Fee – a monthly fee for services like sending statements, disbursing loan payments, etc.

You can learn more about HECMs online at HUD.gov.

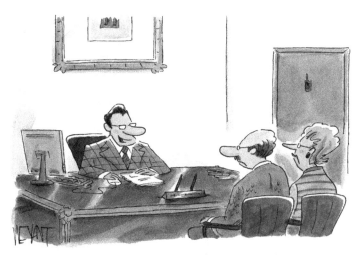

"Of course, you can always supplement your retirement income with panhandling."

FIVE FINANCIAL FIXES FOR SENIORS

- Embrace senior discounts.
- Revisit your budget. Unless you're independently wealthy, you may have to cut back on some wants to make sure you can cover your needs.
- You don't have to support your kids once they reach adulthood. If they're healthy, they should be able to support themselves. Besides, it may prevent you from ending up in the poor house (sorry if we sound overly *Dickensian*).
- Find a cash-back credit card that suits your needs and use rewards for big-ticket necessities.
- Make your money work for you. The worst place to keep it is in a savings account with a low yield. Find a safe alternative: CDs with higher rates, money market accounts that pay higher returns than traditional savings accounts.

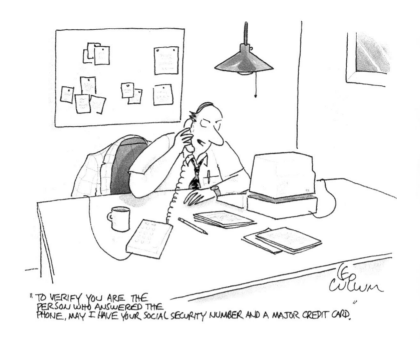

"TO VERIFY YOU ARE THE PERSON WHO ANSWERED THE PHONE, MAY I HAVE YOUR SOCIAL SECURITY NUMBER AND A MAJOR CREDIT CARD."

SENIOR SCAMS

"The oldest, shortest words, yes and no, are those which require the most thought." —Pythagoras

They called me on the phone, and the deal sounded so good, I couldn't say "No!" And then they robbed me blind. So, you ask, "Why Seniors?" The answer is they're easy targets because they are:

- More trusting and polite.
- Have accumulated more savings.
- May not monitor their credit cards as closely.
- May not be tech-savvy.

Scams come in all shapes and sizes: phone calls, emails, or posts—direct to the consumer. It's an easy credit card steal.

- Experts say most victims of scam abuse are females, while males are more often the perpetrators.
- According to the Senate Committee on Aging, almost three billion dollars are scammed from seniors annually. And the Treasurer Inspector General for Tax Administration says, approximately 2.4 million Americans have been targeted by IRS impersonators at a loss of $72.8 million.

Common scams include:

- IRS calls. They are the number one scam. Remember, the IRS does NOT make phone calls.
- Computer support scams are also common.
- Calls about "loved ones in trouble."
- Foreign lottery tickets.
- The Federal Trade Commission says telemarketing scams are the most common contact method against seniors.

Online romance is yet another type of scam. So be careful and don't fall in love so fast.

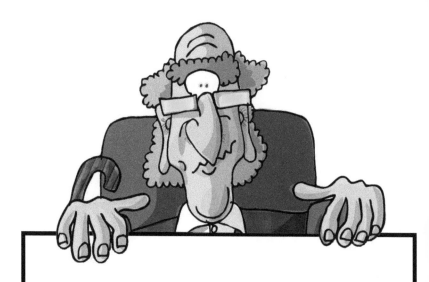

"It's good to be here…
but at 98, it's good to be
anywhere."

—George Burns

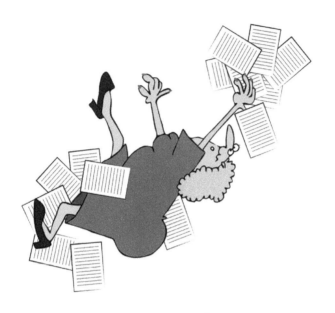

That's
Entertainment!

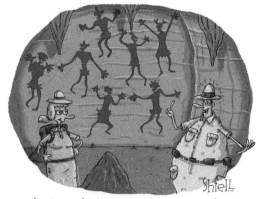

Anthropologists discover the earliest
known depiction of Jazz Hands.

AND THE TONY GOES TO...

Creativity does not retire just because you're over sixty. Take a look at this list of Tony winners:

1. Dick Latessa – 72 – *Hairspray*
2. Cicely Tyson – 89 – *The Trip to Bountiful*
3. André De Shields' – 73 – *Hadestown*
4. Elaine May – 87 – *The Waverly Gallery*
5. Annette Bening – 60 – *All My Sons*
6. Laurie Metcalf – 63 – *Hillary and Clinton*
7. Bryan Cranston – 63 – *Network*
8. Jeff Daniels – 64 – *To Kill a Mockingbird*
9. Beth Leavel – 63 – *The Prom*
10. Fionnula Flanagan – *77 – The Ferryman*
11. Kristine Nielsen – 63 – *Gary: A Sequel to Titus Andronicus*
12. Mary Testa – 63 – *Rodgers & Hammerstein's Oklahoma!*

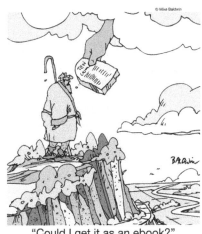

"Could I get it as an ebook?"

FOURTEEN BOOKS WITH OLDER PROTAGONISTS

1. *Murder at the Vicarage* - Agatha Christie
2. *Operation Underpants* - Mark A. Briggs
3. *Mrs. Palfrey at the Claremont* - Elizabeth Taylor (no, not that Elizabeth Taylor)
4. *The 100-Year-Old Man Who Climbed Out the Window and Disappeared* - Jonas Jonasson
5. *The Lido* - Libby Page
6. *Three Things About Elsie* - Joanna Cannon
7. *The Little Old Lady Who Broke All the Rules* - Catharina Ingelman-Sundberg
8. *The Unlikely Pilgrimage of Harold Fry* - Rachel Joyce
9. *The Thursday Murder Club* - Richard Osman
10. *Olive Kitteridge* - Elizabeth Strout
11. *News of the World* - Paulette Jiles
12. *Mr. Loverman* - Bernardine Evaristo
13. *The One-in-a-Million Boy* - Monica Wood
14. *90 Lessons to Learn From a 90-Year-Old: Wit and wisdom from author and actor David Leddick* – David Leddick

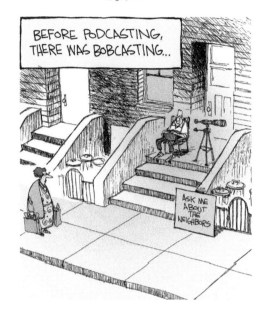

RADIO PODCASTS GEARED TOWARD OLDER PEOPLE

- Health and Well-Being
    www.wcbs880.radio.com
    Host: Pat Farnack

- Stuff You Should Know
    www.howstuffworks.com
    Hosts: Josh Clark, Charles W, "Chuck" Bryant

- Planet Money
    www.npr.org
    Host: Jacob Goldstein

- Criminal
    www.thisiscriminal.com
    Host: Phoebe Judge

- This American Life
    www.thisamericanlife.org
    Host: Ira Glass

- Ask Me Another
    www.npr.org
    Host: Ophira Eisenberg, Jonathan Coulton

- Stuff You Missed In History Class
    www.podcasts.apple.com
    Hosts: Holly Frey, Tracy V. Wilson

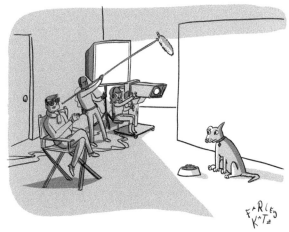

"Your motivation is that you're a dog and it's food."

AND THE BEST DIRECTOR OSCAR GOES TO...

What we said to introduce the Tony awards holds true for the Oscars.

- Clint Eastwood – 74 – *Million Dollar Baby* (2005)
- George Cukor – 65 – *My Fair Lady* (1964)
- Martin Scorsese – 64 – *The Departed* (2007)
- Carol Reed – 62 – *Oliver!* (1969)
- Roman Polanski – 69 – *The Pianist* (2003)
- Jane Campion – 67 – *The Power of the Dog* (2021)
- Kathryn Bigelow – 58 – *The Hurt Locker* (2010)
  (Yes, she was only 58, but she's the first woman ever to win an Oscar in the Best Director category.

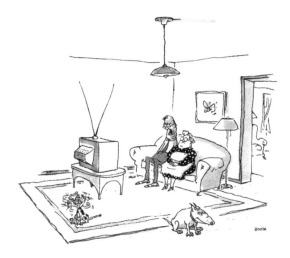

"I just now dreamed I was in bed watching TV."

FIFTEEN TV SHOWS THAT FEATURE OLDER PEOPLE

1. *Grace and Frankie*
2. *Blue Bloods*
3. *Hot in Cleveland*
4. *Downton Abbey*
5. *Off Their Rockers*
6. *$h*! My Dad Says*
7. *Murder She Wrote*
8. *Forever Young*
9. *The Golden Girls*
10. *The Kominsky Method*
11. *Matlock*
12. *The Good Place*
13. *The Good Fight*
14. *Barry*
15. *Better Late Than Never*

"We don't stop playing because we grow old; we grow old because we stop playing."

—George Bernard Shaw

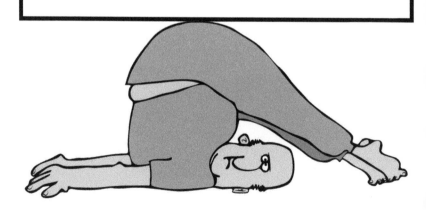

Board Games For People Your Age...
1. Poops and Bladders
2. End of **LIFE**
3. Bunions and Dragons
4. Badbackgammon
5. Apples to Apples Dust to Dust
6. Gasword
7. Clue-less
8. Operation (and rehab)
9. Sloppily
10. Ants in the (stretch) Pants

and...

GAMES PEOPLE PLAY

Games have been around for thousands of years. Board games have been around the longest, 5,000 years. If we look back in history, we will find many of the games we play today have been around for centuries; tile games and rolling the dice, to name a few. Think craps.

Games have always been an important part of our daily lives. They bring people together and enhance our social life. They can be competitive and cause our adrenaline to spike and create excitement. And games can be learning tools to keep our minds sharp by helping enhance our mental health and cognitive skills. This is especially important for the senior population since we may not be as sharp as we once were. (Ask my daughter, she will attest to that). Our brains need to be stimulated. For me, getting out of bed and facing the day is my first challenge.

So, get ready. Pick a playmate, a challenger, or just relax and play online word games by yourself.

All games have a purpose. And they're fun.

- Concentration–It's a card-matching game to try and improve your memory. I played that a lot as a kid. But I still don't remember why the hell I went into the kitchen.
- Card games–Canasta, Gin or Gin Rummy, Go Fish, and Bridge. Cards are social and strategizing. And if you like War, it's good for reflexes.
- Video Games–Not just for kids. It's just plain fun. You can play it solo or invite competition.
- Word Games–My favorite of all. Scrabble, Words with Friends, Wordle. Competition at its finest; thinking, strategizing, increasing your vocabulary.
- Outdoor Games–tennis, pickleball, bocce, shuffleboard. Good physical activity. It helps with eye-hand coordination.
- Chess–Planning ahead, strategizing, and it's great for the brain.
- Crossword Puzzles–Challenging, relaxing, and a great learning tool. Use a pencil.
- Jigsaw Puzzles (for when you just need to go to pieces).
- Arts & Crafts–Challenge your imagination. Maintains hand and finger flexibility.
- Brain training apps–Available to download. They say these apps improve visual, concentration, and problem-solving skills.

It's always the right time to improve your memory, so put the pedal to the metal and let the games begin!

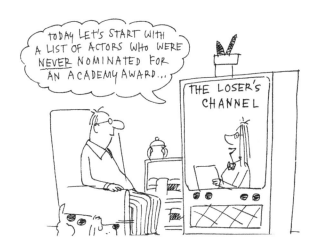

AND THE OSCAR GOES TO…

You don't have to be a spring chicken to win an acting award:

- Christopher Plummer – 82 – *Beginners* (2012)
- George Burns – 80 – The Sunshine Boys (1975)
- Henry Fonda – 76 – *On Golden Pond* (1982)
- John Wayne – 62 – *True Grit* (1970)
- Jack Nicholson – 60 – *As Good as it Gets* (1998)
- Paul Newman – 62 – *The Color of Money* (1987)
- Jeff Bridges – 60 – *Crazy Heart* (2010)
- Peter Finch – 60 – *Network* (1977)
- Katharine Hepburn – 74 – *On Golden Pond* – (1982)
- Jessica Tandy – 80 – *Driving Miss Daisy* (1990)
- Meryl Streep – 62 – *The Iron Lady* (2012)
- Frances McDormand – 60 – *Three Billboards Outside Ebbing, Missouri* (2018)
- Marie Dressler – 63 – *Min and Bill* (1931)
- Geraldine Page – 61 – *A Trip to Bountiful* (1986)
- Helen Mirren – 61 – *The Queen* (2007)

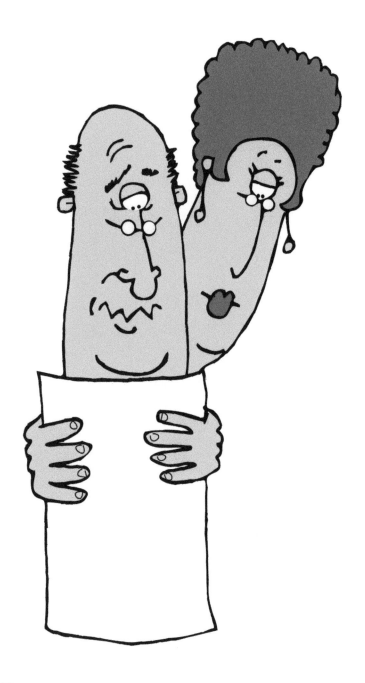

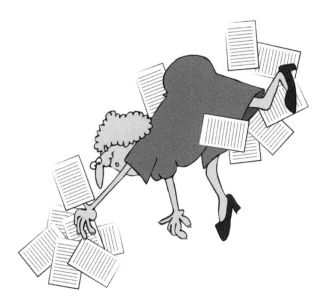

Travel
Virtuosity

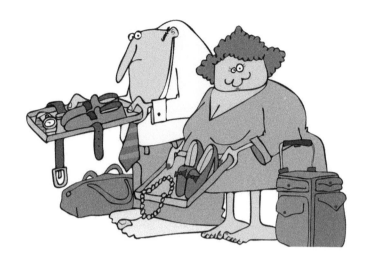

BEFORE YOU GO GLOBETROTTING

- Contact your health care provider to see if you need vaccinations, booster shots, or prescriptions.
- Make a list of the medications and supplements you need to take with you.
- Make a list of contact information of your health care providers to take with you.
- Make a list of current health problems and treatments.
- Consider buying travel health insurance with pre-existing illness coverage (if needed).
- Many cruises have easy, moderate, and difficult levels of excursions. Choose wisely.
- Discuss any physical/health limitations with a travel agent. Some tour organizers cater to senior travel.
- Look online for medical facilities in the places you're visiting.
- Read a guidebook and make a plan before you go.

- You may want to get a dental checkup before you go. No one wants a toothache at 40,000 feet.
- Only take the one or two credit cards you plan to use and contact the issuer about your travel plans. I once had my credit card denied in Copenhagen because the bank thought the charge was fraudulent.
- Arrange to have local currency for the first country you are traveling to. After a canceled connecting flight, we once had to hire a taxi in Switzerland to take us to a different city to catch a riverboat before it sailed. We didn't know until we arrived at our destination that the driver would only accept cash and not credit cards. It was several hundred euros. Luckily, we were able to cover the fare.
- Consider wearing a medical alert pendant or bracelet overseas. (And this is just to go to New Jersey.)

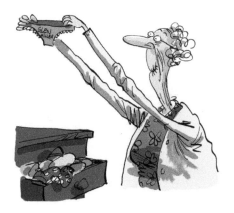

PICKY PACKING PERFECTION

Just a few tips about luggage and what to put in it.
Carry-on:

- Pack medications in their original Rx containers along with a copy of the prescription.
- You may want to pack a spare pair of prescription eyeglasses.
- It never hurts to pack a small first aid kit containing Band-Aids, moleskin (for blisters), antiseptics, antacids, and painkillers.
- Pack jewelry or other small valuables you couldn't bear losing in your carry-on.

Checked luggage:

- It's easier to use a suitcase with wheels.
- Don't overpack; learn to coordinate.
- Keep your checked luggage receipts handy.

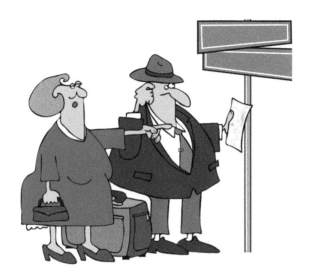

ON THE RUN TRAVEL TIPS

- Wear compression stockings to avoid developing clots in your legs (deep vein thrombosis).
- Wear loose, comfortable clothing.
- Avoid alcohol.
- Avoid sitting with your legs crossed (unless you have to pee).
- Perform leg and foot stretches.
- Don't try to do too much. Arrange for plenty of downtime.
- Don't sit for too long. Take frequent breaks so you can get up and walk.
- Use hand sanitizer frequently.
- Drink plenty of water. However, if you're in another country, don't drink any water that doesn't come in a sealed container.
- Avoid ice cubes in other countries. Your gastrointestinal system will thank you.
- Always wear seatbelts.
- Don't ride a motorcycle. If you must, wear a helmet.

- Know local traffic laws before you drive.
- Ride only in marked taxis.
- Avoid overcrowded or top-heavy buses and vans.
- Pay attention when crossing the road in countries where they drive on the opposite side of the street.
- Don't travel at night.
- Don't wear expensive jewelry.
- Consider carrying a dummy wallet with a small amount of cash in case you're mugged, or use a money belt under your clothing.

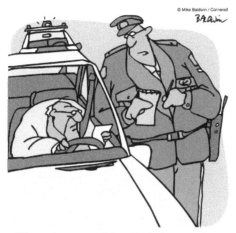

"If you have to drive that slow, put on your emergency flashers to warn other drivers. Or better still, wear a hat."

YOU'RE DRIVING ME CRAZY!

Probably one of the toughest decisions we will have to make as we get on in years is when, or if, we should stop driving. It's been a great ride for us and the more than 45 million drivers over the age of 65, according to the CDC.

Hardly any 60-plussers we know ever want to stop driving. It's literally our key to leading an independent life.

But as we age, the probability of getting into accidents increases. Depressing thought, I know, but there are ways to ensure our safety and the safety of the other drivers. These tips apply to all age groups, but who doesn't need a refresher course? However, if all else fails and you find yourself getting into more fender benders, perhaps the time has come to call an Uber.

So, what's a driver to do?

- We know the obvious—don't drink and drive. Wear your seat belt, and don't drive in lousy weather.
- Get your eyes and ears examined regularly.
- Don't drive at night if the glare from oncoming cars affects your vision. You can, however, purchase anti-glare glasses. My husband uses them and feels more secure.
- Don't become distracted by your cell phone. Not easy, I know. Maybe turn it off.
- Know the directions beforehand. Changing lanes at the last minute is not a good idea.
- Remain physically active. Simple motions like turning your head or looking over your shoulder can be challenging if you're stiff.
- Don't tailgate. You should be at least two car lengths behind the car in front of you.
- Don't get behind the wheel if you're nervous.
- Make sure your medications don't interfere with your concentration or physical abilities.
- Listen to your family members and friends when they tell you to hand over the car keys.

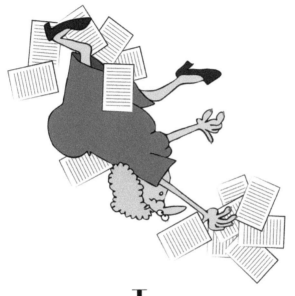

In
Closing

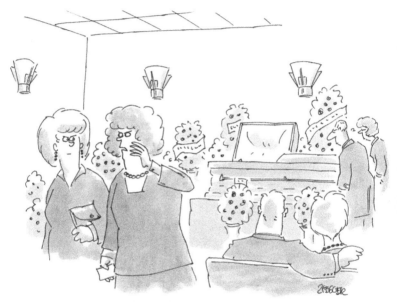

"Well, finally! Gracefully aging no more."

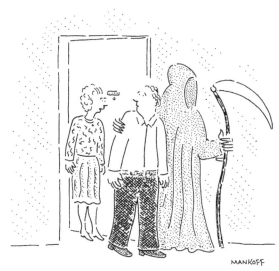

"Relax, honey—change is good."

SAYING "GOODBYE" IN ELEVEN LANGUAGES

Arabic	Mae al Salama
Bengali	Bidāya
French	Au Revoir
German	Auf Wiedersehen
Hindi	Alavida
Israeli	Shalom
Japanese	Sayōnara
Mandarin	Zàijiàn
Portuguese	Adeus
Russian	Do Svidaniya
Spanish	Adiós

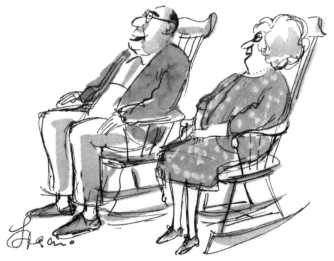

"Because of you, my darling, I've never had an ulcer. I've never needed a psychiatrist. When I poured out my troubles, you listened. When I ranted and raved, you listened. Thank you, my angel, for listening."

"Who listened?"

IN GRATITUDE

During uncertain times, many of us try to harness our fears and emotions while feeling totally out of control. Our thoughts become unhinged as we imagine the worst-case scenarios.

To stop the noise, take a breath. Concentrate on what you have… not what you are afraid to lose.

Hanging on the wall in my office is a simple sign that says, "Acceptance." It's just one word that carries with it so many emotional descriptors. And when I look at that word, I feel a sense of calm because of the message it carries. On the other side of that list is my gratitude list. I created it when the pandemic sliced into our lives, rendering us helpless. On the other hand, I felt so very lucky that we were spared the ravages of what this virus has done to so many and may continue to do.

You can call your list whatever you like. The main focus is to reign in positivity.

Whatever you feel grateful for, write it down. These are some of mine, which I add to when necessary.

- I am grateful for my family.
- I am grateful for my daughter, who yells at me when I slip up.
- I am grateful for my rescue dog, Coco, who brought us so much joy.
- I am grateful that I have a roof over my head.
- I am grateful that I have a computer.
- I am grateful I have the friends that I have.
- I am grateful for my friend and co-author, Carol. Together we have created this book, among others. And I love her.
- I am grateful that I hear birds chirping in the morning.
- I am grateful for my morning coffee.
- I am grateful that I survived breast cancer and hope to continue to do so.
- I am grateful that I have a best friend I trust with my life.
- I am grateful that I have food on the table.
- I am grateful that at my age, I'm only a little hard of hearing.
- I am grateful that spring has sprung, and I see the buds of new life.

My co-author's list is much shorter—like she is—but like her parrot, she will repeat many of the items that are on the above list. She just can't help herself.

Here it is:

- I am grateful for my family.

(See, I told you she was going to copy me. Just saying…)

- I'm grateful my husband keeps everything around me running efficiently while I'm locked away in my office, writing.
- I am grateful my little parrot provides comic relief.
- I'm grateful one of my bonsai trees chose to live
- I'm grateful I have a roof over my head.

(There she goes again.)

- I'm grateful I have a co-author who is generous and prolific.
- I am grateful Barbara is only a "little hard of hearing," or else together, we'd be useless.
- I am grateful I have an active imagination that rarely takes a day off.
- I am grateful to every single person who has ever read one of my books and ecstatic if they chose to read more than one.
- I am grateful for the life I have led, full and rich with a close-knit family, wonderful friends, and great co-workers.
- I'm grateful for my cousin, Joann, who is virtually my twin, separated at birth. She's my sounding board and offers excellent suggestions when I'm perplexed.
- I'm grateful I can make the font really big on my iPad, so I can read several novels a week.
- I'm grateful I was able to skip a lot of lines, so my list looks as long as Barbara's.

We are grateful that you're taking this journey with us and hope you enjoyed this *Book of Lists*.

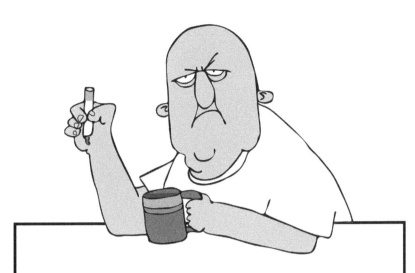

"When I die, I want to die like my grandfather, who died peacefully in his sleep. Not screaming like all the passengers in his car."

—Will Rogers

ACKNOWLEDGMENTS

We would like to thank our editor, Susan Keillor for tidying up our writing. We honed our skills in television newsrooms where people heard our words rather than saw them, so they never truly witnessed our lack of punctuation know-how. Of course, there may still be a few mistakes in this book from thoughts we added after the editing process. (It's *your* job to find them and report back).

Our cover art and several of the non-captioned images in the *Book of Lists* are by Dennis Cox, whose work was purchased through Shutterstock.com

We also want to thank Sean Hanley-Horwood and everyone else at CartoonStock Ltd. for helping us with our insatiable need for funny stuff. Sure, we think we're funny on our own, but maybe not *that* funny. And even though one of us used to be an art major, that talent has crashed and burned as you can witness in the cartoon, below. CartoonStock is *sooo* much better.

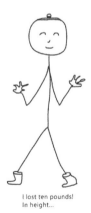

I lost ten pounds!
In height...

(SOMEHOW, THIS TYPE OF HUMOR NEVER WORKS WITH A STICK FIGURE)

You're welcome.

ABOUT THE AUTHORS

Carol Pack and **Barbara Paskoff** are well known for their collaborative works, *Over-Sixty: Shades of Gray, a Journey Through Life's Later Years (On the Road to Fossilization)*, a book about the aging process, *Mind Games & Soporifics*, a puzzle/coloring book, and *Our Coronavirus Diary*, their personal experiences with the travails of dealing with a pandemic.

Carol Pack is an award-winning former journalist, news anchor, assignment manager, college professor, and a former president of the Society of Professional Journalists—Long Island Chapter. During her journalism career, she taught more than a thousand graduate and undergraduate NYIT college students how to get jobs as broadcast journalists at the school's internship, *LI News Tonight*. She also worked as a news writer for WNBC-TV, News 12 Long Island, and GNYC News. She has received numerous awards from various media organizations including the Fair Media Council, New York State Broadcasters Association, the Society of Professional Journalists, and the Press Club of Long Island. In 2018, Carol was inducted into the Long Island Journalism Hall of Fame.

She now has a second career as both a non-fiction author and a novelist that includes a young adult fantasy series known as the *Library of Illumination*. Kirkus Reviews named *Chronicles: The Library of Illumination* one of the best indie books of 2014 and has given a critical nod to each of the subsequent books. She is also the author of the historical fantasy series: *Evangeline's Ghost*.

Carol received both her BA and MA from New York Institute of Technology. A native New Yorker, she lives on Long Island with her husband Andrew and her picky parrot.

ABOUT THE AUTHORS

Barbara Tuerkheimer Paskoff, a founding partner of Envision Productions, Inc., and a former broadcast journalist, has produced and written medical and public affairs programs since 1988 for PBS and cable stations. Her work has been broadcast throughout the United States. She has received four Emmy nominations, as well as awards from the Press Club of Long Island, New York State Broadcasters Association, Long Island Coalition for Fair Broadcasting, the Aurora Award, The Columbus International Film & Video Festival Award, The American Medical Association International Health and Medical Film Competition Award, and the New York Institute of Technology Alumni Recognition Award.

She has written, produced and directed medical education videos for pharmaceuticals, doctors, and patients. She has also served as Executive Vice President of the Society of Professional Journalists— Long Island Chapter. She divides her time between writing, competitive dancing and tennis.

Barbara received her BS from Emerson College in Boston and her MA from New York Institute of Technology. Born in New York, she now resides on Long Island with her husband, Michael.

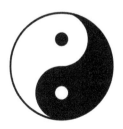